The Medical Professional's *Guide to* Handheld Computing

Chris Helopoulos

JONES AND BARTLETT PUBLISHERS
Sudbury, Massachusetts
BOSTON TORONTO LONDON SINGAPORE

World Headquarters

Jones and Bartlett Publishers
40 Tall Pine Drive
Sudbury, MA 01776
info@jbpub.com
www.jbpub.com

Jones and Bartlett Publishers Canada
2406 Nikanna Road
Mississauga, ON L5C2W6
CANADA

Jones and Bartlett Publishers International
Barb House, Barb Mews
London W6 7PA
UK

Library of Congress Cataloging-in-Publication Data

Helopoulos, Chris.
The medical professional's guide to handheld computing / Chris Helopoulos.
p. cm.
Includes index.
ISBN 0-7637-3152-8
1. Medicine—Data processing. 2. Pocket computers. I. Title.
R859.7.P62 2003
610'.285'416—dc21

2003011835

The author, editors, and publisher have made every effort to provide accurate information. However, they are not responsible for errors, omissions, or for any outcomes related to the use of the contents of this book and take no responsibility for the use of the products described. Throughout this book, the author has used the trade names of devices, software, and documents created by Palm Inc., Sony, Samsung, and many other manufacturers, publishers, and individual or collective software developers. These devices, software, and documents are the trademarked property of the corporations, institutions, or individuals that created or have purchased the rights to them in accordance with United States and international copyright and patent laws. The reader should understand that, although the symbols ™, ®, and © were omitted for convenience by the publisher, the products mentioned in the text are all proprietary and should be regarded as copyrighted and/or trademarked entities. Products and devices described in this book are not endorsed by the publisher, nor are any guarantees regarding their functionality made or implied by the publisher or author.

Production Credits:
Acquisitions Editor: Christopher Davis
Production Editor: Elizabeth Platt
Cover Design: Brianna Donahue
Manufacturing Buyer: Therese Bräuer
Composition: Modern Graphics, Inc.
Printing and Binding: Malloy Lithographing
Cover Printer: Malloy Lithographing

Printed in the United States of America
07 06 05 04 03 10 9 8 7 6 5 4 3 2 1

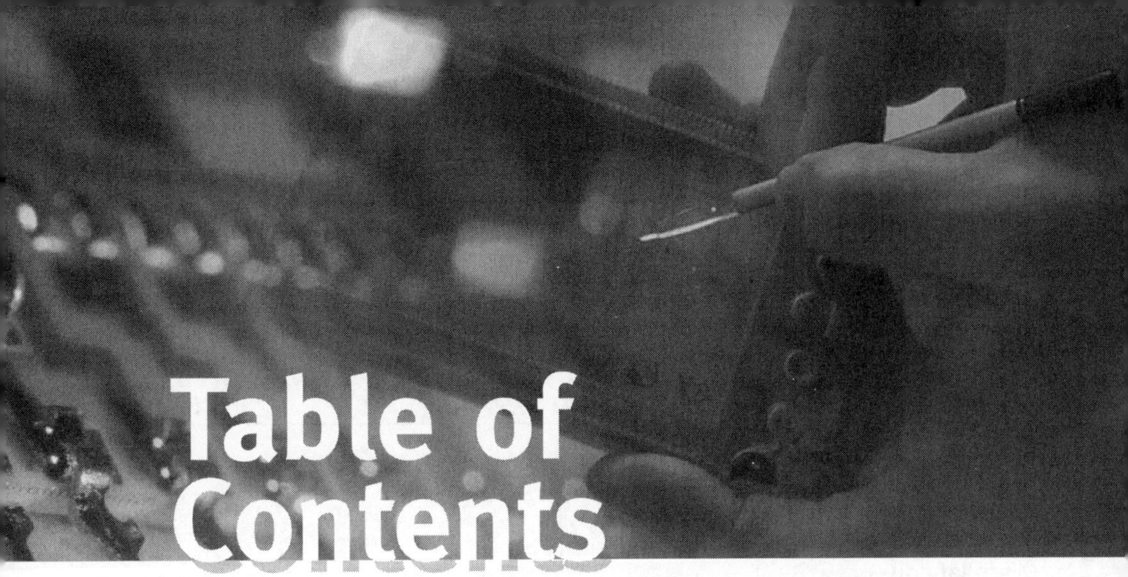

Table of Contents

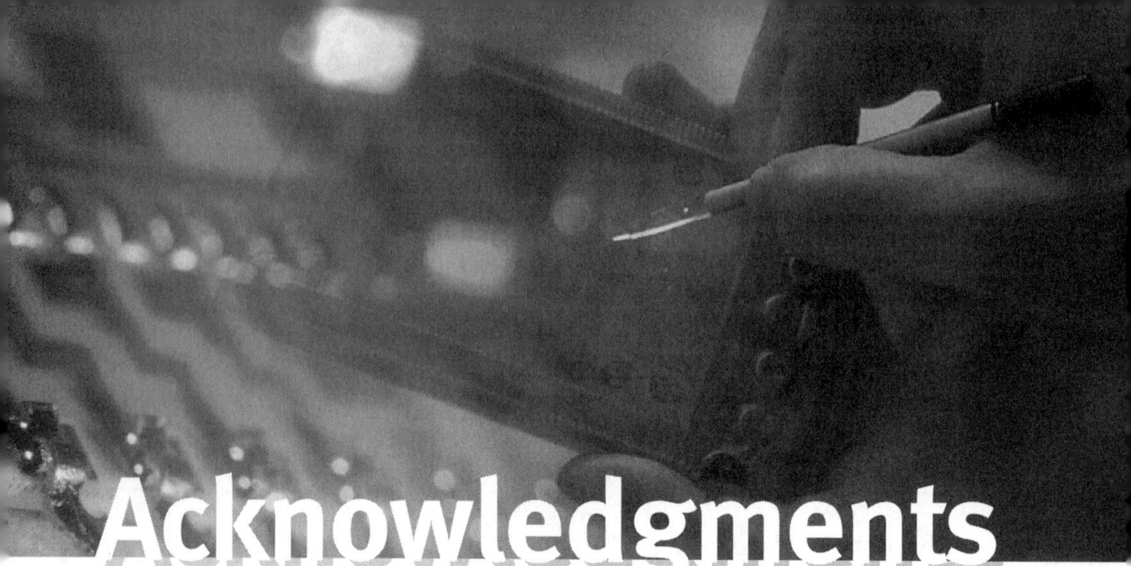

Acknowledgments

Many people have helped to make this book possible. Although I cannot possibly name them all here, I would nevertheless like to offer thanks to a few. First, I thank my colleagues and the administration of Barry University, particularly those involved in the physician assistant program, for their patience and understanding of my single mindedness. They allowed me the flexibility to complete this book. Second, I thank the students of the Barry University Physician Assistant Program, as they were my guinea pigs and field testers. Along the way, they also taught me a lot about handheld computing. Sometimes reluctant, often enthusiastic, they exemplify the range of experience of medical professionals with handheld computers. My friends, family, and colleagues who read, offered suggestions, and gave me insight deserve special thanks. Also, I could not have written this book without the help, input, and permission of a long list of software authors, hardware manufacturers, and corporate entities who made it possible for me to share illustrations and software with you. I owe a debt of gratitude to all of those medical professionals who pioneered the use of PDAs before me. They explored new ground and worked out many of the wrinkles before I ever bought my first handheld computer. Finally, and certainly not least, I want to thank my wife, Terry. Without her gentle giraffe-like nudging, this book would still be a pipedream.

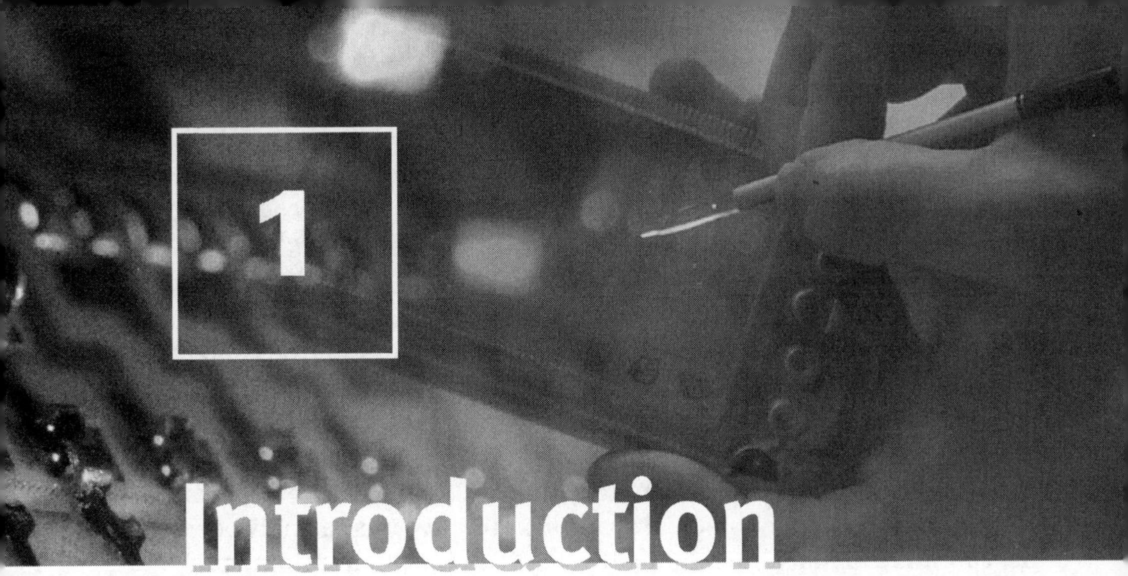

1 Introduction

Welcome to the incredible world of handheld computing in medicine! This book is designed for medical professionals at every level of training, including seasoned professionals. I have sought to make it understandable to the novice in computing, but even the long-time user of handheld computer technology should find something new. If you've been curious about all of the handheld fuss, this book will hopefully answer your questions. If you've been looking for a way to incorporate a handheld computer into your professional practice, this book will help you to realize that desire.

If you're like me, "show and tell" was your favorite tradition in grade school. I liked showing something new or different but was equally fascinated when someone else did the same. Handheld computing is certainly similar. It's the kind of "toy" that we could only dream of as a child, and it's getting better every day. I say toy because that's exactly what my wife thought my first handheld computer purchase would become. She was convinced that it would soon be discarded in a drawer somewhere. Now, more than 3 years later, she can see how indispensable it has become and how I rarely ever put it down. She never brings up that idea anymore since I bought her a PDA; in fact, she has adopted it into her own practice of medicine as a physician assistant.

I, too, am a practicing physician assistant and Associate Director of Clinical Education for the Barry University Physician Assistant

Program. As a student, perhaps along with you, my lab coat pockets were bulging with helpful little handbooks of medicine. We've come far since then. I still have the same desire to have many different medical references at my fingertips, but it has become amazingly easier and technologically more powerful to carry them in a handheld computer. It's a lot more streamlined, too.

In my teaching capacity, I began to wonder whether our physician assistant students might also benefit from this technology. For that matter, couldn't our institution learn a few things from data that our students could gather during their clinical training? Let me add that this was not unique or revolutionary thinking. It was just new for us. Other schools and other medical professionals have increasingly been incorporating laptops and handheld computers into their training programs and practices. As for data gathering, paper surgical logs have no doubt been kept for decades. I just proposed that we skip the paper step altogether. Why not teach our students handheld technology, give them a tool for logging their clinical encounters, let them gather that data and feed it back to us at school, where we can analyze the patient encounter data?

After more than 3 years of this experiment, we've learned a lot. Our physician assistant students have become savvy with their handhelds. During clinical training, they enter each patient they encounter into their handhelds, using software we have developed, in about 1 to 3 minutes per patient. Meanwhile, they have amassed a vast arsenal of medical references to carry with them in their handhelds. We discuss some of it in this book. They've taught us a few things along the way, as well.

We, in turn, have gathered their data, merged it, and analyzed it—rather, we continue to analyze it. We've learned about the demographics of the patients our students see, what kinds of illnesses they have, and what kinds of medical procedures are used in their treatment. This information is valuable in evaluating training sites and equalizing the training for all of our students. What's more, all students will be able to assemble a creditable document detailing the scope, breadth, and numbers involved in their entire clinical experience. This will be invaluable to them for future credentialing.

The background for this book has now been set. Students come to our school with various levels of experience with handheld computers, including no experience at all. Some embrace new technology, and some are fearful of things that they don't understand. Maybe you fit into one or the other of these groups. The idea of this book is to level the playing field. If you don't know anything about handhelds—maybe you're not even sure whether you need one—this book should explain how and why. Maybe you've seen other handheld computer how-to books, but they didn't talk to YOU, a professional in a medical setting. That's the gap that we're trying to fill with this book. Handhelds are useful to a lot of people in many settings, but perhaps no place more useful than in medicine. Medicine has often led technology, and few fields change faster than medicine. This places a tremendous burden of knowledge on medical professionals. This book demonstrates how handheld computer technology can benefit doctors, nurses, physician assistants, and all students of medicine. It will take you from the basic to the specific, and then you can decide for yourself: "How did I ever survive without one before?"

How to Use This Book

It is our hope that a broad range of medical professionals will find this book useful and helpful. It seems appropriate that I include a few notes about how to get the most out of this book. First, I don't want to be negative, but I want to be honest. This is not the kind of book that you are going to sit down and read cover to cover like a novel, as that would surely induce sleep. I think, rather, that you should check the table of contents and skip to a part that is personally relevant. For example, if you haven't yet bought a handheld computer but are thinking about it, then you should consult Chapter 2 before making your purchase. If you just bought a PDA and want to jump into using it, then you should take a look at Chapter 3 (Getting Started). Whether a new user or an old hand at PDAs, you'll want to check out the appropriate software sections.

Second, there is no way that this book could hope to be all-inclusive. A lot of useful information is contained herein, much that has been learned by trial and error, and much that has been gained by spending a lot of time on the Internet. I've tried to touch on everything relevant to a medical professional, but necessarily, some things have gotten more emphasis than others. For example, no substitute is available for reading the instructions that came with your handheld computer. These often go into great detail about setting up, using, and troubleshooting your brand of PDA. Do we always do this? Unfortunately, no. Therefore, I have tried to include a Quick Start Guide for the inevitable impatient practitioner. Similarly, I have generally utilized the Palm OS as the model throughout this book. The reader can infer that much of what is said can also apply to Pocket PC models of handhelds. However, it is best to refer to the original instruction manual to confirm specific points.

Third, feel free to skip around. For example, you may find out about HanDbase in one section (or while surfing the Internet) and decide to add it to your PDA. You might then want to skip to the section in the book that details some of the available medical offerings that you could add to your PDA that work with HanDbase. Another example is in Chapter 7 (Medical Commercial Software). You might find it helpful to read the reviews of all of the Skyscape products together because there is quite a bit of overlap and commonality to the way they work. Similarly, Handheldmed titles will have a lot in common with one another.

Fourth, pick up and put down. Try out and come back. Experiment, read, and experiment again. That's the handheld computing experience. A PDA is undoubtedly a computer, but it's a tool nonetheless. You didn't just pick up a stethoscope and suddenly know how to use it. You had to play with it, use it, and get familiar with it. It wouldn't do just to read about a stethoscope. PDAs are like that too.

Finally, use the resources contained in the book as a springboard. This book is a starting point. I've tried to include web sites, companies, and titles that will lead you to further exploration. To that end, we have included a very useful CD-ROM. With this tool inserted into your desktop computer, you will be able to go easily to various PDA web sites without having to type in the web address. You will also be able to install free software and trial/demo versions of commercial software more easily to your PDA because we have included them on the CD-ROM. I hope that you find your handheld computer to be as indispensable to your practice of medicine as I have found it to mine. May this book launch you into a lifetime marriage of handheld technology and medicine. I welcome your comments and suggestions for future editions. Feel free to contact me at chelopoulos@mail.barry.edu.

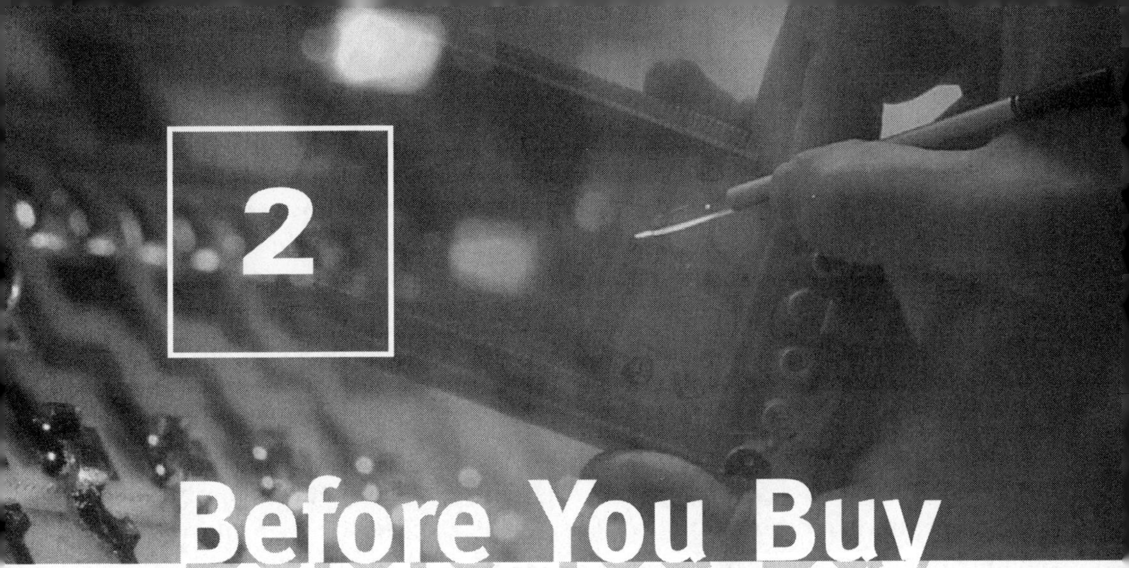

2 Before You Buy

Assessing Your Needs

It may be difficult to assess your handheld computer needs at this stage (when you're new to handhelds), but ultimately this is what you should do before you actually make a purchase. If you're new at this, you may want to explore some of the features and capabilities of handheld computers first and then assess your needs. If you're more experienced with handhelds, maybe now would be a good time to reevaluate what you want to accomplish with your device.

In the simplest and most basic way of looking at a handheld computer, it has historically been called a PDA or Personal Digital Assistant. In the earliest models, apparently all that was envisioned for the device was a means of transferring some crucial data from the desktop computer to a portable device that you could carry with you. These types of functions are still some of the most vital and basic tasks expected of today's handhelds (e.g., maintaining a date book and a phone book). These items are hard to leave behind at the office. The handheld computer not only makes the office version portable, it allows you to make changes on your handheld while you are on the go; these changes are later synchronized to the office desktop computer, thereby saving duplication of effort. All of today's devices perform these functions extremely well. If this kind of activity is your basic need, you'll be satisfied with even the lowest priced model of handheld.

Many medical professionals and others need the availability and portability of reference materials. Again, handhelds come through with excellent performance, and once again, even the lowest priced models perform splendidly. The ability to display text is built into every handheld computer, but as is discussed in a later chapter, it is dependent on software to accomplish the task. If your need is a handy reference tool, any handheld will do nicely, and your attention later turns to which software to add to your device to help accomplish this task.

Other needs may not be as basic. If you want your device to be used primarily for the input of information, you'll be more acutely aware of input methods and options. We'll discuss these in more detail later, too. Basically, the question is this: Will you become comfortable with and adept at stylus input, or will you rely on keyboard entry? If the latter, should your device come with a built-in keyboard or have the capacity for an add-on keyboard? Similarly, we explore such needs and options as telephones, wireless Internet connectivity, and more.

Thus, the more that you know about handheld computers before making the purchase decision, the more likely you will be to make a rewarding purchase. With this being said, don't set your expectations too high by expecting the handheld computer that you purchased today to be your final purchase for many years. Devices are changing and improving rapidly, and thus a great model today is likely to be eclipsed in performance and features by tomorrow's model, often at an even lower price. Moreover, your needs may change or increase as your use of the device increases. What you expect out of a handheld computer today is not very likely to be what you expect out of one in the future. My point here is not to complicate the purchase decision-making process with a plethora of details but to assure you that it is normal, perhaps even desirable, to "trade up" in a year or two.

Shopping and Comparing

One of the most rewarding things for me is "the hunt," the chase to make the right purchase and "catch" the right price. Often people are afraid of making the wrong choice, afraid of buying the "wrong" model or the wrong brand. This is a perfectly natural feeling. When you're new to this, it seems as if a dizzying array of choices are available. That's because there are! The best way to feel more confident in your choice is to be better informed. Here are a few tips that you can try.

1. Scour the electronics ads. Retailers commonly advertise all of their specials in flyers that are inserted in the Sunday newspaper. I review these religiously each week to see what's new and what's hot. Shop and compare.

2. Talk to other handheld computer users. Although it may be true that every person owns the "best" PDA, they may also be able to tell you why they selected that particular model, what features they like the best, and what model they prefer today and why. Filter their views in the context of what it is that YOU want, what's important to YOU.

3. Try before you buy. Haunt the electronics stores and try the various models. Many stores have a knowledgeable sales staff in their PDA departments, who don't just steer you to the most expensive model without showing you the features of each model.

4. Check out the Internet. All of the major handheld manufacturers have web sites that are loaded with information on all of their models—usually with the retail prices and sometimes with demonstrations of key features. Try www.company_name.com (e.g., www.handspring.com) to get to most sites. Sites of larger companies may take a little more navigating once you get there (e.g., click on their consumer electronics section and then "handheld computers").

5. Know that it's a buyer's market right now. We are getting more for less, as all of the electronics companies are battling each other for our dollars. In the process, most brands have strikingly similar features and capacity if you compare similarly priced models from competing companies. The bottom line is this: It's HARD to make a bad choice.

6. If all else fails, feel confident that if you're not completely happy with the model you've chosen, it's not the end of the world. It's a relatively small-ticket purchase, and

something better will likely be available in just 6 months. When the urge gets overwhelming again, buy a new PDA and give the old one to somebody you really like!

Hardware Options

Operating System: Palm versus Pocket PC

The operating system (OS for short) is the biggest initial difference between PDA models. Just as Windows or Macintosh is used for your personal computer (PC), the handheld comes with a built-in OS. For our purposes here, the OS is either "Palm" or "Pocket PC." Remember that these are operating systems only—not brands. Several competing brands use the same OS. If your PDA uses a particular OS, it is compatible with any other PDA using that OS, even if it is another brand. For example, our students use the entire gamut of Palm, Sony Clie, and Handspring Visor brands because they all use the Palm OS. This enables them to share programs and information between models even if they don't share the same cords or other hardware. Compare apples to apples.

For the most part, cross-connectivity is not possible between models with different OSs. This means that if you have a PDA that uses Palm OS, you basically will not be able to beam information or share programs with another user who has Pocket PC OS and vice versa (this is not universally true but is a pretty good generalization). Some notable exceptions exist, and often software comes in both versions. For the most part, however, consider the two OSs as separate species.

A few months ago, I would have said that your choice of OS depends on what you want to do with your handheld. I no longer think this is true. Such advances have been made recently that I feel you could probably accomplish the same tasks with either OS. Aficionados of either OS can give you innumerable reasons about why their particular brand of OS is best. Pocket PC users often point to the easy interconnectivity between Microsoft PC functions (word processing, calendar, address book, etc.) and their handhelds. Add to that the attractive fact that Pocket PC models have often been multiuse devices incorporating MP3 players, color picture viewers, voice recorders, and so forth into their hardware, and you begin to get an idea of what attracted the Pocket PC buyer in the first place. Palm OS is the more established OS and has attracted a loyal following because of ease of use and programming as well as lower cost, generally. What's more, newer Palm OS devices tend to incorporate more of the fancy multiuse features that were once exclusive to Pocket PC devices, so the chasm that once separated them is now narrowing.

So, which OS should your PDA have when you shop for it? In the current marketplace, I think there are two important considerations. First, which of the OSs are your colleagues using? If you are in a group practice, for example, and it's important for the various clinicians to be able to share information between PDAs, then you'll want to make sure that their OSs are compatible. It will be much simpler if everyone is using the same OS. Again, this does not necessarily mean the same brand or model, just the same OS. Second, and probably the most important point, which OS offers the software choices that you need? Although this may be changing, I believe that the Palm OS currently offers more software for medical professionals. We'll look in depth at software later.

Internal Memory and Expansion Memory

Low-priced or entry-level models of some brands may have fixed memory limitations. More models are coming out with memory expansion capabilities. You wouldn't think of buying a PC today without a CD-ROM drive. If you get a PDA without expansion capability, that's exactly what you're getting. Don't misunderstand me, a basic PDA has its place; in fact, it may be the carrot that gets you into this PDA game. However, be assured that today's sufficient memory will soon become tomorrow's woefully inadequate memory. For a variety of reasons, internal memory beats add-on memory and add-on memory beats no memory expansion capability whatsoever. Just think ahead and buy the most memory you can afford. You'll be grateful soon.

Monochrome versus Color

Someday all PDA screens will likely be in color, just as PCs are now. Meanwhile, color screen models generally continue to be pricier and notorious hogs of battery life. I'm beginning to see the benefits that color brings to some applications, such as icon recognition and game playing. Software developers can do a lot more with color than they can with grayscale on a monochrome screen. In addition, a color screen has better visibility in darker areas (e.g., patients' rooms). Programs are generally written to work on both color and monochrome models. Alternatively, they may come with two versions, and you install the one for your kind of handheld. The future promises both lower power consumption color screens and also better batteries. All in all, color is just more impressive when somebody is looking over your shoulder. I have always considered the color models a luxury, but now that they have come down in price, I'll likely give in soon.

Batteries versus Rechargeable

This seems like a small point, but consider it up front. Built-in rechargeables may cost a bit more, but you'll save in the end. Some models, such as the color ones, eat up power and are more likely to come with built-in rechargeables. Mine is a monochrome model with built-in rechargeables. I get good life out of a recharge and like the convenience and reassurance of simply plugging it in. Consider whether this is an important feature. We discuss later, in Chapter 3, that battery failure causes a catastrophic crash and loss of data. Therefore, whichever choice you make, keep an eye on your battery charge 0status.

Other: Wireless, Keyboard, Multifunction (Phone)

Similar to internal memory and expansion memory discussed previously in this chapter, handhelds come in two flavors with regard to their Internet capability. Wireless PDAs have an added feature that allows the user to access the Internet and check e-mail without being connected to a computer. Of course, this comes at a price and requires payment of a monthly service fee to activate that wireless service. Currently, this is at least $20 per month. Other than that one function, wireless or wired, most PDAs do the same things. Also, consider that depending on the model that you choose, it may be possible to add on wireless capability with some additional third-party hardware. Ask in advance and research the accessory first. Although I see looming potential, I am personally taking a wait-and-see approach to wireless.

Also, handhelds now come with or without built-in keyboards. Those without built-in keyboards can likely use one of a variety of third-party add-on keyboards. Therefore, your options are quite wide. Consider how much data you are likely to input, how comfortable and adept you are likely to become with stylus (Graffiti) input, and how portable you want to be. For many users, Graffiti is all that they need and want. For others, the tiny built-in "thumb" keyboards are the ideal solution to data input. Personally, I have never been very adept at inputting large amounts of Graffiti with the stylus. I prefer the popup keyboard screen for most of my input. When I have more text to input, I like the full-size add-on keyboard, which is reviewed later. In that case, I am giving up portability for speed of entry.

The next option that you might want to think about before buying your handheld is a cell phone. In the past, this was not a consideration, but it's now important. Several choices are available, but basically one must decide whether to buy a phone with a built-in PDA or a PDA with a built-in phone, or whether the two should ever be combined at all. There are distinct advantages to each. With the widespread and ever-growing use of cell phones and the growing adoption of PDAs, it is easy to see why the predictions are for more of the so-called convergence devices that combine the capabilities of both into one device. It has been a boon to me to have one less item to carry and to have the convenience of a PDA that is also my cell phone. Impressive features can also be incorporated when you marry two devices like this. It is no wonder they are often referred to as "smart phones." It is beyond the scope of this book to go into all of the features of phones incorporating PDAs or PDAs incorporating phones. Once more, you should shop and compare, keeping the OS in mind at the same time.

Brand and Model

Other features are too numerous and varied to list. These are the subtle features that differentiate PDA models just as facial features differentiate people. Hold PDAs in your hand to feel which is potentially more comfortable. Look at screens in bright and low light. Check out backlighting features, controls (like jog-wheel thumb controls), built-in keyboards and flip covers, and software that comes with the PDA. Look, touch, feel, try, compare, and consider their usefulness or importance to you.

3 Getting Started

Quick Start Guide

My best advice is, of course, to read carefully the instructions that come with your handheld computer. My PDA came with a setup disk that included a complete electronic manual. These instructions are usually well thought out, with basic step-by-step procedures and more advanced troubleshooting. I still refer to mine periodically when I encounter a problem. However, I also know that many new purchasers, students, and medical professionals want to turn their devices on and start playing with them right away. For you, I include the following Quick Start Guide.

Setup

After unpacking your handheld, the first step is to supply it with power. Install fresh batteries properly if your model requires them or charge the internal rechargeable batteries if your model comes with them. When that is done, turn on your device. When the device is turned on for the first time, a picture animation walks you through the first steps (Figure 1). Don't ignore these important first steps.

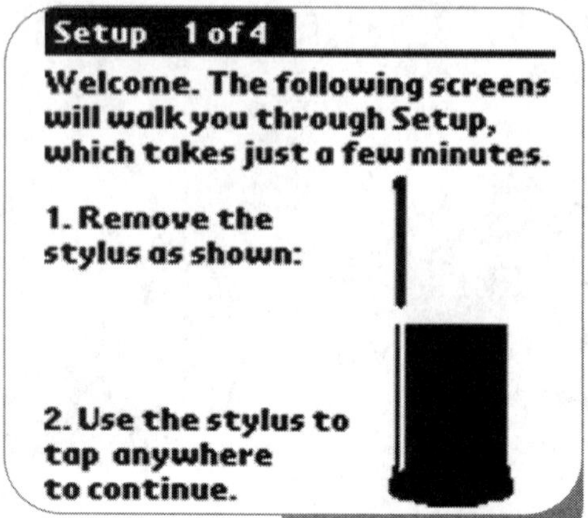
Setup 1 of 4
Welcome. The following screens will walk you through Setup, which takes just a few minutes.
1. Remove the stylus as shown:
2. Use the stylus to tap anywhere to continue.
Figure 1

You will see a series of small "targets" (Figure 2A) that you are asked to chase around the screen with your stylus. This is the digitizer, which helps your device to pinpoint where you are actually writing later with the tip of your stylus. New users have come to me in the past unable to figure out why their device seems inaccurate or unresponsive to the touch of their stylus. The answer is that they didn't take the time to use the digitizer properly. This can be corrected later, but it is easier to do it right the first time.

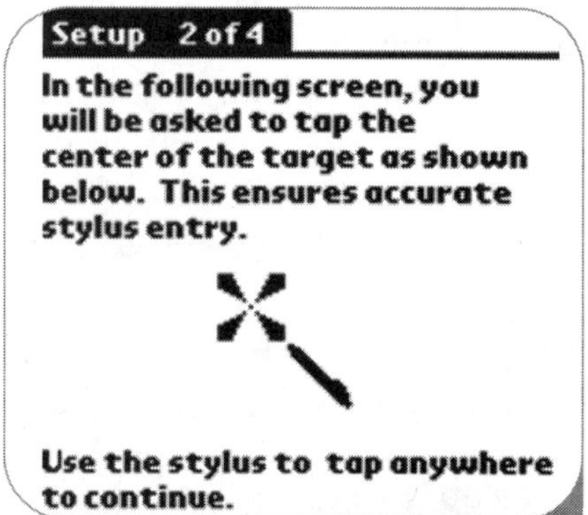

Figure 2A

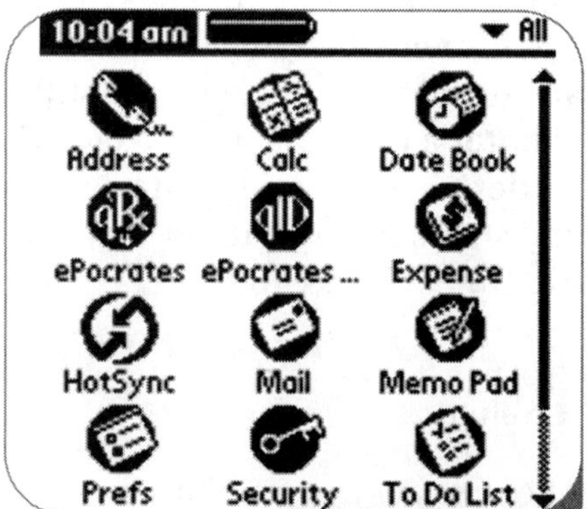
10:04 am
All
Address
Calc
Date Book
ePocrates
ePocrates ...
Expense
HotSync
Mail
Memo Pad
Prefs
Security
To Do List
Figure 2B

You should then see the "launch" screen (similar to that shown in Figure 2B). From here, tap "Prefs," which will take you to the Preferences page (Figure 3A). Although you could skip this now and come back to it later, it is where you choose some of your personal preferences for sounds, set the time and date, and so forth. All of these actions are simple and are initiated by tapping on the screen in the respective area with your stylus. Whenever you see an arrow, tap on it to reveal a "dropdown" menu of choices. If you tap on the choice you want, it becomes highlighted and will become your setting when you move on to the next item or exit. Time and date are similarly set by tapping on their dotted-line boxes to reveal choices to select by tapping with the stylus.

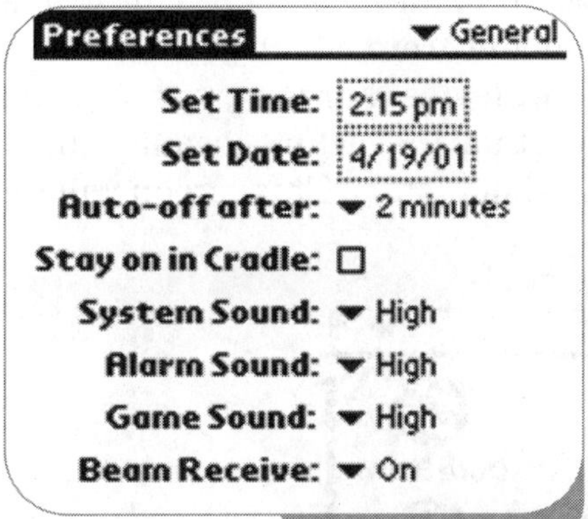

Figure 3A

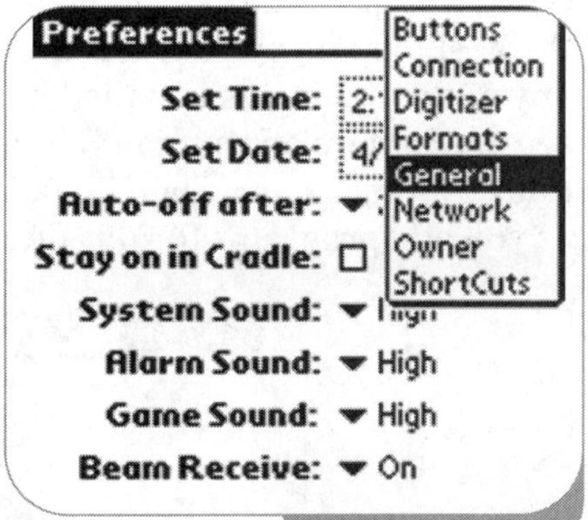

Figure 3B

Notice that "General" in the upper right-hand corner of your screen (Figure 3A) has an arrow that always means dropdown choices. Tap on this arrow and the dropdown menu shown in Figure 3B will be displayed. Tap "Buttons" to see the screen shown in Figure 4.

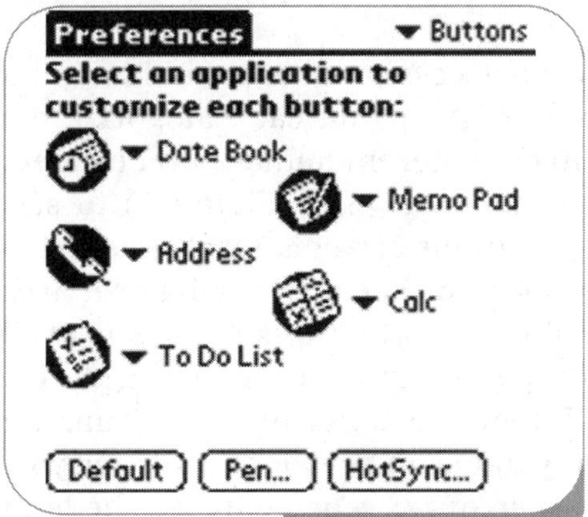

Figure 4

Here you can choose what functions to assign to the various buttons of your device. You can keep the factory (default) settings or reassign the functions that open on your handheld when you press different buttons. These can be changed at any later time, too.

Exit Preferences by tapping on the Applications or Home icon. This varies by device but will be a flat, internal, printed (also called "silkscreen") button that is built in to your device and is located just left of the Graffiti box area. We'll call this the Launch icon. When you tap it, a display similar to that shown in Figure 5 is seen. This is like the desktop on your PC. It is the launcher from which you can enter any of the programs installed on your device. For now, you may not see much more on your launch screen than the factory-installed functions (Address Book, Date Book, and Calculator). This screen will fill as you add programs to your device.

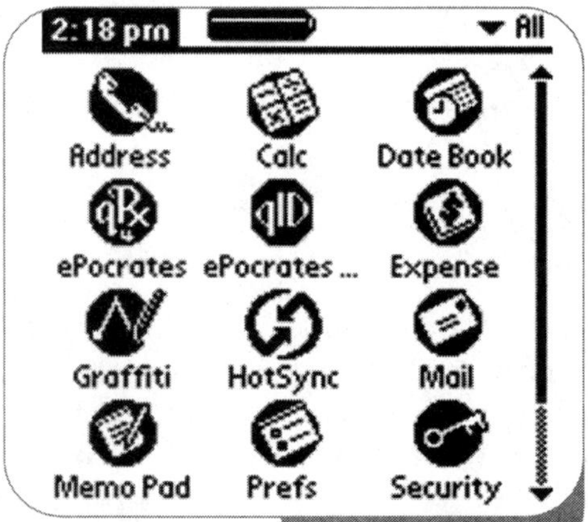

Figure 5

Note that you can access some items either by button or from the launch screen. In addition, you can categorize items to find them more conveniently in different launch screen categories. Tap on the dropdown arrow that says "All" (Figure 5) to see the other categories to which programs are currently assigned. You can reassign them and/or create new categories, whatever works best for you. For now, it's good to know that this feature is available. Also, keep an eye on that dropdown arrow in the top right-hand corner of the launch screen. When you think that programs have disappeared, chances are that you haven't selected "All" for your launch screen. Use the dropdown arrow or repeatedly tap the launch icon to make this happen.

Another important button is the Menu (silkscreen) button, which is just below the Launch button. Tap on it to see a display similar to the one shown in Figure 6.

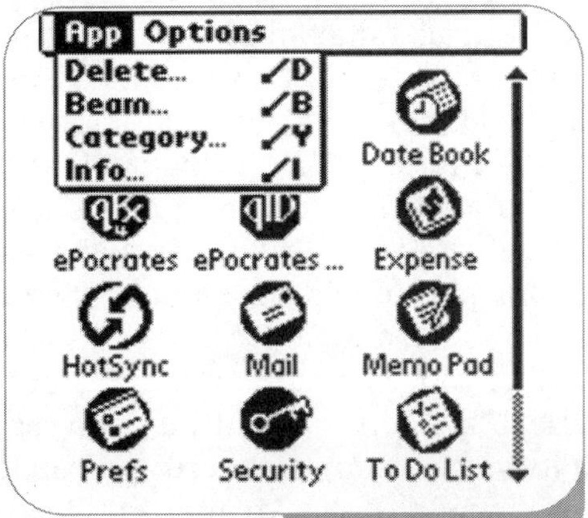

Figure 6

From here you can select information to view about all of the installed individual programs (e.g., their size and version, and to which category they're currently assigned). You can also decide whether to delete individual programs or to beam them by infrared to another user. The options choice allows you to set preferences for your launch screen (basically, whether icons should be large or small). At other times, when you are in a specific program (not the launcher program), the menu button takes on other functions. Use it to explore the program that you are using, its features, options, preference settings, and copyright and registration information. When you want to know more about a specific program that you have opened, tap on the menu icon.

HotSync

HotSync is the name given to the synchronization that is performed between your PDA and your PC. This is such an important function that it could be compared to the umbilical cord in utero. You could basically use your PDA right out of the box without having attached it to your desktop PC for a HotSync. At some point, however, it will become necessary for your PC to communicate with your PDA and vice versa. They do this through the HotSync process. Why is this necessary? Several reasons exist.

HotSyncing allows the user to move vast amounts of information between the two devices, thus eliminating much duplication of effort. For example, all of the contact information you have on your PC (e.g., addresses, phone numbers, and other important information that resides in Microsoft Outlook, for example) can easily be copied to your PDA at HotSync. This saves a lot of time and insures better accuracy than re-entering the data by hand. You might also find it convenient to enter new contacts into your PDA while out of the office. You'll be comforted to know that at HotSync these new entries can be designated to synchronize with your desktop data and will be seamlessly integrated with your previous desktop data. The same is true for your Calendar, Memo List, and To Do List. This is a real time saver and insures that all of your most important data are with you whenever you need them. If you don't currently use Microsoft Outlook, your PDA comes with its own desktop software and can accomplish all of the previously mentioned tasks by keeping duplicates of the PDA entries on the PC desktop version.

However, HotSyncing has additional benefits. Eventually you'll want to add software to your PDA. Whether you purchase a CD-ROM or download the software from the Internet, the software goes to your PC first, allowing you to keep a copy of the software on your PC. The way the software is installed on your PDA, however, is by HotSyncing the device to your PC. This allows you to install the new software from your PC to your PDA. This happens very quickly while contacts and other data are being synchronized.

Finally, one other very important reason for HotSyncing is for BACKUP. Each time you HotSync your handheld device, a backup file of all of your data and programs is created on your PC. This is invaluable insurance against loss of your PDA, accidental damage to the device, or the inevitable crash (and accompanying loss of data). Frequent backups can save you countless hours of data reentry and are worth scheduling on a regular basis. Crashes occur occasionally, and they always occur when you least expect them and have the most data to lose.

Various models will have variations on the theme, so you should refer to the product instruction manual to become familiar with this process, although we do review the basics here. Your PDA came with an installation/setup CD-ROM. Besides usually including a thorough instruction manual, this disk includes the desktop software for your PC. Run this disk on your PC and follow the step-by-step instructions on installation. It will ask whether you want to make Microsoft Outlook your default synchronization to your PDA or whether you want to install the Palm Desktop to your PC. It will ask you whether you want to synchronize your e-mail to your PDA. It will also ask you to choose a HotSync user name for your PDA. This is important because more than one PDA can be synchronized from the same PC, and, in turn, you can synchronize your PDA to more than one PC. Either of these situations can easily arise in the office setting with multiple users. At any rate, pick a user name for your PDA, something simple but unique, that will become your permanent HotSync user name (it is case sensitive).

Now, either attach your PDA to your PC via a plug-in cord or place your PDA into a HotSync cradle that is attached to your PC by a cord. Depending on the make and model of your PDA, these can be either serial port or USB connectors. If you have a cradle, just press a button on the cradle to initiate HotSync. If you are using a cord, tap the HotSync icon from your device's launch menu. When you tap this icon, the screen shown in Figure 7 will be seen on your PDA. Tap on the two arrows icon in the middle of the screen to begin HotSync. When connected to a PC for the first time in either of the previously mentioned cases, the PC will ask whether this is a new PDA user account. This is where you type in your HotSync user name the way you want it to appear. Your new HotSync user name will eventually appear in the upper left-hand corner of your PDA screen. In Figure 7, my HotSync user name is "DEMO."

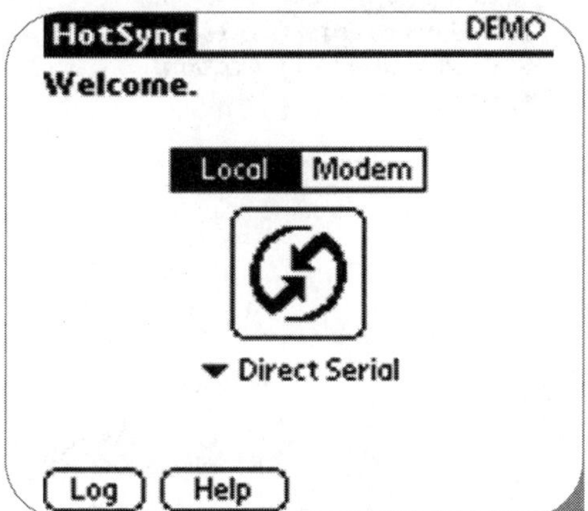

Figure 7

HotSyncing is as simple as that. Nuances certainly exist beyond this simple basic process, but we won't go into them in depth here. Refer to your owner's manual for further details about making choices as to whether, at any given HotSync, the handheld data should override the desktop data or vice versa. You can make these choices separately for each of the four basic functions (address book, calendar, memo list, and to do list), and you can decide whether these settings should be default settings or temporary. All of this is done with the HotSync menu of the Palm Desktop on your PC. Step-by-step instructions are included on your setup disk.

Graffiti versus Popup Keyboard

When you want to make an entry or add data of some sort to your handheld computer, several options are available. Let's say, for example, that you want to write yourself a memo. First, press the Memo hard button (on most models it is the button in the lower right-hand corner that looks like some sort of spiral notebook). This brings up a screen similar to the one shown in Figure 8. Memo will be displayed in the upper left-hand corner, and the screen will show a list of the existing memos. The ones shown here are often automatically installed on your device upon first HotSync, just to demonstrate the feature. At any rate, if you want to make a new memo entry, tap New in the lower left-hand corner of the screen (Figure 8).

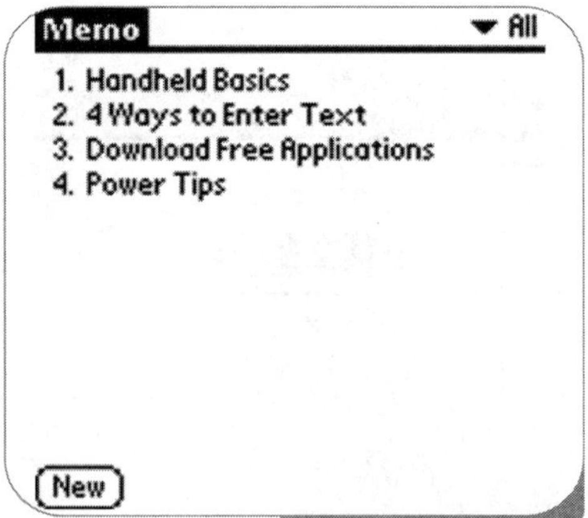
Memo
▾ All
1. Handheld Basics
2. 4 Ways to Enter Text
3. Download Free Applications
4. Power Tips
New
Figure 8

This will bring you to the screen shown in Figure 9. Now you should see the cursor (the small upright line) flashing at the top of the first memo line. In order to start a new memo, the cursor must be flashing. If the flashing cursor is ever missing, just tap where you want it to be flashing. Now you can enter copy for your memo via the simple and quick Graffiti method. That is, you write with your stylus in a stylized alphabet called Graffiti, which your PDA recognizes and interprets as letters. However, don't write your Graffiti up on the screen where the cursor is flashing. Although that's where the copy will end, your device only recognizes Graffiti when it is written in the proper Graffiti area, which is the shaded area of your device's screen bordered by the silkscreen buttons (the Home, Calendar, Calculator, and Find buttons). Enter letters in the left portion and numbers in the right portion.

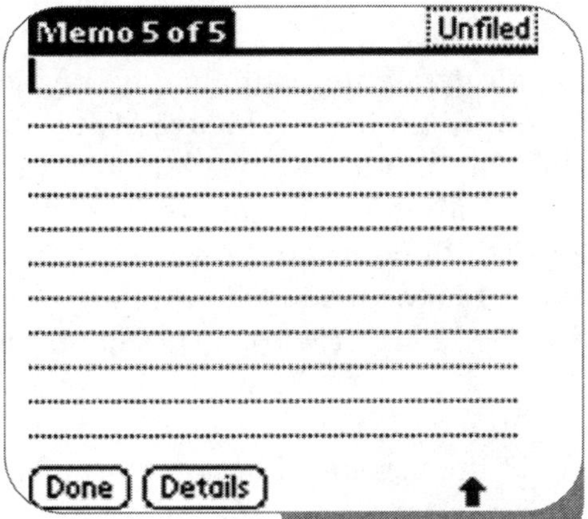

Figure 9

The details of the Graffiti alphabet are not discussed here, but your instructions likely came with more details and a tutorial. Practice certainly makes perfect in this case. If you ever need a quick reference for Graffiti characters, just drag your stylus from the bottom of the Graffiti writing area to the top of the handheld's screen. When you do, you will see a reference screen that looks like what is shown in Figure 10.

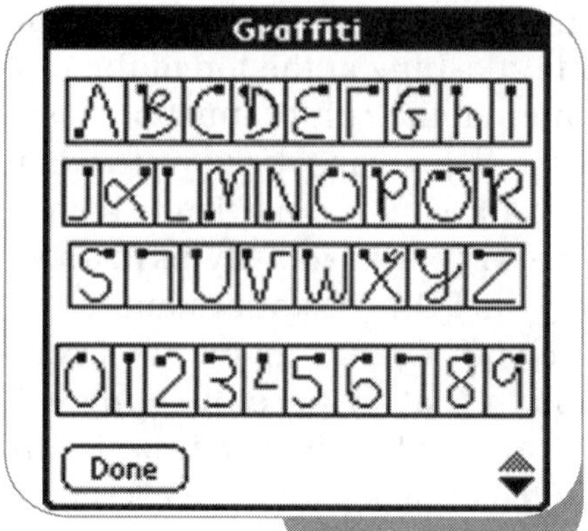

Figure 10

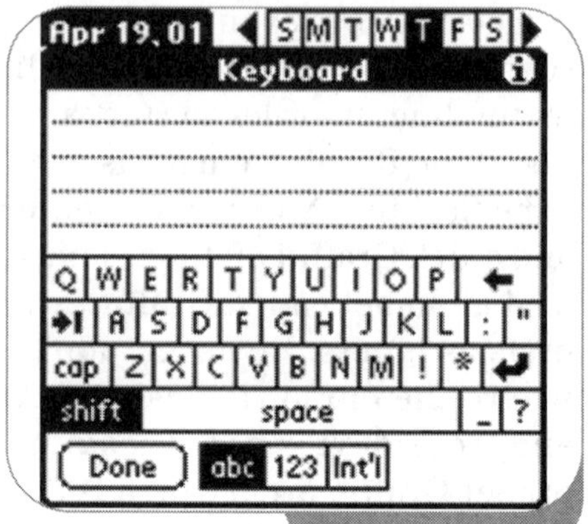

Figure 11

Many users insert a majority of data on the go with Graffiti, as it is easy and portable. You can become quite adept at it in a short amount of time.

Another option for data entry is the popup keyboard that is a feature of your PDA's built-in software. Figure 11 shows one such screen. In this case, we are attempting to make a calendar entry. Similar to what we did with the Memo entry, press the Calendar button (usually the lower left-hand button on the device). Then tap on the date for which we wish to make an entry. This time, instead of using Graffiti, use the popup keyboard (Figure 11). Tap on the "abc" letters in the lower left corner of the Graffiti screen to make the keyboard pop up. (Note that Sony models access the popup keyboard via a small icon in the lower right of the screen). For some brands, you will see that the keyboard is for letters only and is arranged in the familiar "QWERTY" layout of a typewriter or computer keyboard. You can shift to capitalize the next letter (Figure 11), switch to all capital letters, and add punctuation, spacing, etc. The small arrow backs up and erases one space at a time, and the longer curved arrow is like a return or enter key that moves your cursor to the next line of copy.

Try tapping on "123" in the center to go to the number keyboard shown in Figure 12 (the one shown here was accessed while making an entry to the To Do list.) You will see that the numbers are arranged in calculator fashion and that quite a few symbols and punctuation marks are included in this keyboard view. You can switch back and

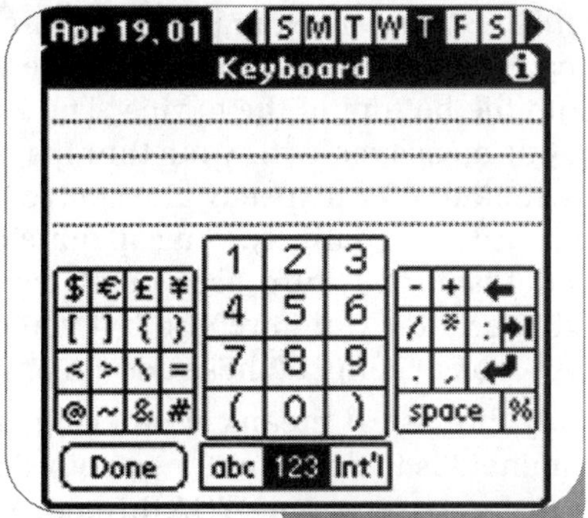

Figure 12

forth between letters and numbers just by tapping the appropriate square of the respective keyboard. In addition, it should be pointed out that the number keyboard could also be accessed immediately from the Graffiti screen (anytime you have a flashing cursor) by tapping the "123" area of the Graffiti screen, just as we tapped the "abc" area in the first place (Figure 12).

These illustrations have shown screen shots that are common to most of the Palm OS devices (e.g., HandSpring and Palm brands). More recently, I have noted an improved keyboard (one that combines alphabet and numeric keys on the same keyboard) on Sony Clie devices using Palm OS 5. I don't know whether this is inherent in the new Palm OS. For those of you without benefit of the new keyboard, we see later how you can upgrade yours with a small software addition.

I personally find the popup keyboards to be the most comfortable and familiar to use. I imagine that I am giving up some speed by not perfecting my Graffiti skills, but I seem to find things more readily when using the keyboards. For me, punctuation, spacing, and symbols become important, and these seem a bit more confusing in the Graffiti system. You may be different, however; thus, spend a little more time practicing Graffiti, and you may find that it suits your needs.

These are not the only means of entering data into your handheld. You may have decided that data entry on the go was going to be a major use of your device. In that case, you may have opted for a model with a built-in pushbutton keyboard, which increasingly is being offered on more models. Current examples of this are the HandSpring Treo and the latest Sony Clie NX models that have a small "thumb" keyboard built into the bottom of the device. The keyboard is operated by pecking out messages with your thumbs as you hold it in your hands. This should offer a speedy alternative to either Graffiti or the popup keyboard. Alternatively, you can quite likely add one of a growing number of "add-on" (third-party or aftermarket) keyboards to your handheld later after you purchase it if you determine that's what you need. We look at some of these add-on options later.

Finally, probably the fastest means of entering large amounts of data into your handheld is to do the entry on your PC or laptop computer and then transfer it over to your PDA through a HotSync. Large-volume memos, to do lists, addresses, or calendar entries can be easily handled this way. Later we talk about software for transferring other data to your PDA.

Cautions

It is prudent to advise you of a few early caveats to help in preventing some of the more common pitfalls. We learn from our mistakes, but maybe a few words to the wise can save a little frustration.

Batteries

Thou shalt not let thy batteries run completely out. This is such a serious error with such catastrophic consequences that you're not likely to let it happen a second time. Your handheld computer probably has a low-battery warning feature built in to its software. If you see this warning, take heed because if you lose power, you lose everything. When you restore power, your device will look like it did with the factory installation. All data and other programs that you have installed will be lost. Your only hope of recovery is your backup file on your desktop PC or other backup devices, to be discussed later. Individual programs can be reinstalled individually, but data are painful to reinstall if you have not backed up recently. Don't let your batteries run down! Keep fresh batteries on hand or recharge your rechargeables frequently to insure that this doesn't happen to you. If it does, you'll be sorry.

Backup

As you may have guessed from the previous battery caution, you should make a habit of backing up your handheld device, as this takes only a few minutes but is worth the time. By backing up, of course, we mean performing a HotSync between your handheld and your desktop PC. This should be a regular exercise, whatever is a safe pattern for you, but probably at least weekly. Why? Because backing up insures the protection, the archiving, of your data. It can synchronize data both ways, whether added to your handheld or added to your PC. It insures against more than battery failure, too. There are other causes of major handheld "crashes" necessitating resets and the resultant loss of data. These devices aren't foolproof. Also, your handheld could be lost or stolen, which is bad enough, but a loss of valuable data would be even worse. The bottom line is this: Back up frequently and regularly. Make it a good habit from the start.

Scratches: Styli, Screen Savers

The screen, which is the window through which you view everything on your handheld, should be treated carefully. Although it's not exactly fragile, it's certainly not bulletproof either. It is certain that you'll have your screen as long as you have your device. Scratching it will be like looking through dirty glasses for the rest of your ownership. This can be prevented by adopting a few simple habits in the beginning. First, use the stylus for tapping and writing on the screen, as it was made for this purpose and will protect the screen in the process. Nearly anything else is tougher on your screen and can potentially damage it. Don't use a pen or pencil on the screen, and avoid touching it with your fingers, too. Clever stylus replacements are available, some with added features. Some pens now come with built-in optional styli. Whatever you choose, make it a tool that was designed for the job of scrawling on your screen without damage. Another option that many users choose is to apply screen savers, which are thin films of clear material that were expressly made to apply over the screen. The idea is that with use you will scratch the screen saver rather than the screen. This works nicely, too. When the screen saver is sufficiently scratched, peel it off. Then throw it away, and apply a new one. At a modest cost, it's worth the investment rather than having to replace the entire screen or handheld device later because of damage.

Cases

Nothing protects your valuable handheld computer better than a good case. These come in every imaginable style, size, shape, and color, with very clever features. As if that weren't enough, I'm aware of at least one web site where the manufacturer even allows you to design your own case. Your handheld probably came with some sort of case. This is a good starting place from which to decide what works best for you. Get in the habit of using it for now. Then decide what other features you might like. The important thing is that the case protects the screen from scratches and blows. It protects the entire device from such things as the occasional drop to the floor, too. Don't think that it can't happen! More than once, I've been saved by a good case. It doesn't necessarily take a drop or a blow to cause damage. A handheld that is squeezed too forcefully in a suitcase, in a briefcase, or between books could also sustain damage. Also, don't forget that the weather can play havoc on electronic devices. A good case can shield your PDA from the weather, too. Because cases are such an individualistic and personal thing, shop around to check them out. How you use your device will help you decide which style works for you. Some people prefer a book-style case that opens and may have pockets or other associated note pads. Others prefer a hard-shell case or a flip-top protector. Some people carry their devices in a bag or pocket. Others prefer to wear their handheld computer using some sort of holster-like case worn on the belt. Will you usually be sitting down with your handheld or attaching external peripheral devices to it? Will you often be accessing it quickly while standing? Do you carry a briefcase or bag that has a good spot in it for your device? These are the kinds of questions that you must ask yourself. In the end, just protect your device with an appropriate case. It will be a good investment.

Insurance

Perhaps the ultimate protection for your handheld computer is extra insurance or an extended warranty. Although I have not purchased this option for any of my previously purchased handheld devices, it seems like it would be a good idea in some cases. Talk to a knowledgeable salesperson and read the fine print before you sign, but an extended warranty could be a lifesaver for some people. One of my colleagues is on his third handheld due to breakage. Students have come to me with cracked screens that need to be replaced. Some retailers' extended warranties actually cover such breakage. Without such coverage, the cost to replace a screen might be enough to drive you to buy a completely new device. Again, shop around and read before you sign. You usually have only one shot at purchasing such extended warranties, which is at the time of purchase.

Basic Built-in Functions

A few basic functions come built in to most handheld computers. These functions are so essential to most users that I think any manufacturer would have an unmarketable product without them. In fact, in most handheld models, the Address Book, Date Book, Memo Pad, and To Do List are four functions that are considered so vital that they are the default settings for the four "hard" buttons. This means that these functions can be accessed rapidly by simply pressing their respective buttons without even turning on the PDA first. A unique feature of these four functions is that they are synchronized to the Palm Desktop at HotSync (or to Microsoft Outlook or a third-party software). Many people, not just medical professionals, use these basic functions. As you will see, however, the basic built-in functions can be very useful in the healthcare setting too.

■ Address Book

One of the two most basic functions of the handheld computer is to serve as an address book. This certainly hearkens back to those early days when the handheld was first called a PDA. What could be more useful than installing all of your sales contacts into your PDA's memory to be retrieved when needed at the touch of a stylus? Well, it's still a vital function today. People on the go do not want to be cut off from their contacts. Also, our contacts are reachable in even more numerous ways than they were before, and we need access to all of those ways. For example, someone might reach me by phone at home, at the office, or en route by cell phone. They could also send a fax (either location), send an e-mail (either location), or even overnight a package to me at either location. Therefore, in order to be complete, somebody's address book entry for me would require at least nine separate pieces of information, as well as my name and title. Handhelds can handle all of this and more.

Press the Address button on your handheld (usually one of the lower left buttons and usually with some sort of telephone symbol on it) to have the address book open. Tap "new" at the bottom of the address book page to open up a page for a new entry. The new entry page will look like Figure 13. First, you'll see in the upper left-hand corner that this new entry will be classified as a business entry unless we choose a different classification. This will become important later if we decide to look at a particular category, for example. Just tap on the dotted-line "Business" box to reveal the other categories, change categories, or edit the types of categories available. Tap somewhere else outside of the box to make the dropdown box disappear. Then you'll see "Last name" highlighted and the cursor blinking at the start of the "Last name" entry line. If the cursor is not blinking, just tap on "Last name" or the "Last name" entry line until it blinks. Whenever you see the blinking cursor, your entry will be made at the point at which you see the cursor, just like on your PC. Currently, you make those entries on your PC by typing on its keyboard. With your handheld, it's even easier. You scribble right on the device's screen. Depending on the model, you may also have the option of inputting your entry with a built-in keyboard. With other models, you have the option of using an add-on keyboard. However, for now, we just want to concern ourselves with this Address book entry. As I have said, data will be placed where the cursor is flashing. You still have to write the entry in the proper Graffiti area of the screen if you are going to hand write it. New users quickly get used to the fact that you don't write your Graffiti right at the point of the blinking cursor.

Similarly, you will go down the page making entries as appropriate for your new contact. "Title" could be Dr., Mr., Ms., or a business title, or you could skip it altogether if it's not applicable. Remember that dropdown arrows mean more choices. Tap on the arrow next to "Work," and you'll see that the first number listed could be reselected to be anything that you choose. This is important because the first position number will be the first number to be displayed. Fill in the rest of the entry lines as applicable to finish the page and even spill over onto the next page (for the same

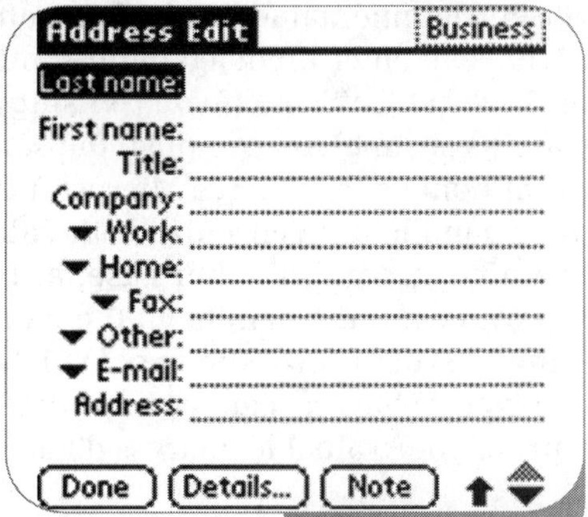

Figure 13

contact) by tapping the arrow in the lower right of the screen. Also, see that you can affix a note (or many subsequent notes) to this contact's entry. You might want to list the contact person's favorite hobbies, for example, or their next of kin. Tap "Done" in the lower left of the screen to make your entry complete. It will automatically file itself alphabetically in your Address book. This is great for when you're away from the office.

Press the Address book button on your handheld to open the address book, and tap on a specific contact's entry to open up the Address View of that contact. This can be displayed in a number of font options by tapping the "Menu" button (lower left-hand corner of your handheld's screen) when in the Address book. I prefer the bold, or middle, choice. Smaller typefaces fit more information to a page, but larger ones are easier to read. Experiment to see what works best for you. The beauty is that you can change the setting whenever you want. The "Menu" button reveals other choices as well.

However, the Address book function is beefier than that. It synchronizes flawlessly with your desktop PC at the office. Not only will the entry that you just made duplicate itself in the PC's address book, but also entries made in the PC's address book will be transferred to the handheld as well with the next HotSync operation. If you've just purchased a handheld computer and have an office PC that contains an address book of hundreds of names, you're just beginning to appreciate the possibilities. If you have the good fortune of already having those office entries maintained with Microsoft Outlook, you're in luck. You won't have to enter them again into your handheld. You can move them all over at HotSync. If you're using something else, third-party software likely might accomplish the same thing. If your PC at the office or at home doesn't have Microsoft Outlook, you can choose to have your handheld synchronize with Palm Desktop upon HotSync. This is a nice option. In either case, at HotSync you can have your desktop overwrite the handheld, the handheld overwrite the desktop, or simply synchronize the two. Whichever option you choose, remember my previous caveat: Backup often to avoid the possibility of losing any of your valuable address data.

Date Book/Date Book+

Probably one of the single most useful functions of the PDA—certainly the one that I refer to every hour or so—is the Date Book or calendar function. I simply do not know how I was able to organize my life before I had one of these devices. Depending on your device's software, some version of the following Date Book views is available: the Day, Week, Month, and List views.

Figure 14 shows the basic Day view that starts with nothing listed on the date. Currently, 8:00 a.m. has been selected. Tap there once again to make an entry at that time. Note that this is Thursday, April 19, and that you could easily tap on another day of the week. You can also move forward or back one week at a time from the day that you have selected by tapping on the arrows to the left or to the right.

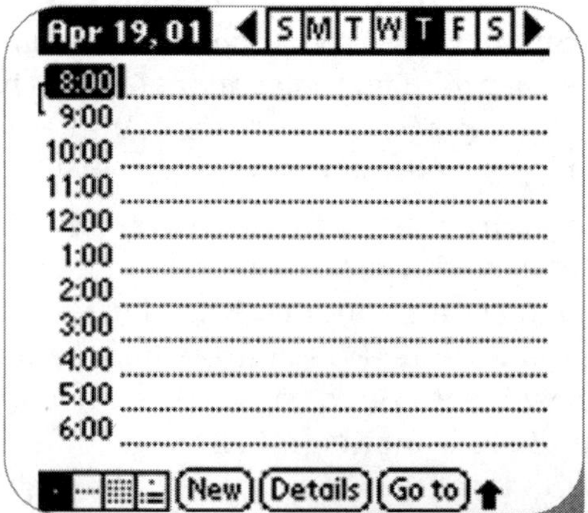

Figure 14

Let's tap on "F" at the top to make some entries for the next day. You'll see the same basic screen as shown previously, but now let's tap "New" at the bottom to make a new entry (Figure 15).

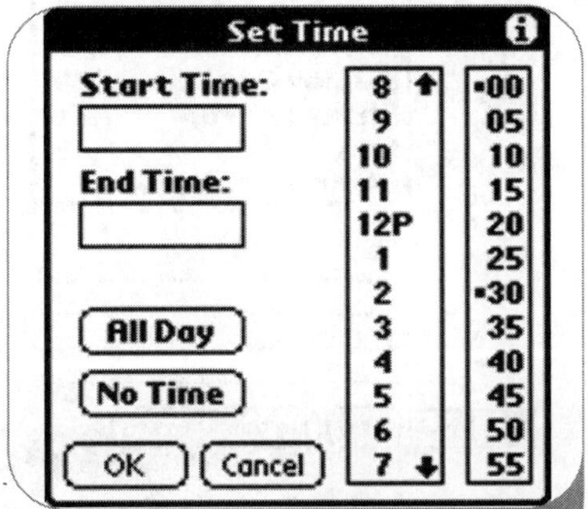

Figure 15

To set an entry with a start time of 8:00, tap on the "8," tap on an end time, or go with the default setting of 1 hour and then tap "OK." Other options would be to make an entry that lasts all day or simply a reminder or untimed event that has "No Time" at all. We can make several entries, and the screen would look like what is shown in Figure 16.

These are just sample entries that illustrate what you can do with your PDA. Be sure to tap the Menu silkscreen button to reveal all of

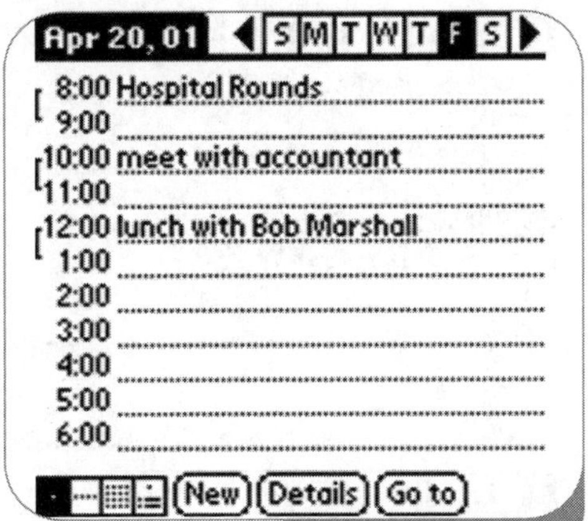

Figure 16

the other options and editing features that are built in to your Date Book function (Figure 17).

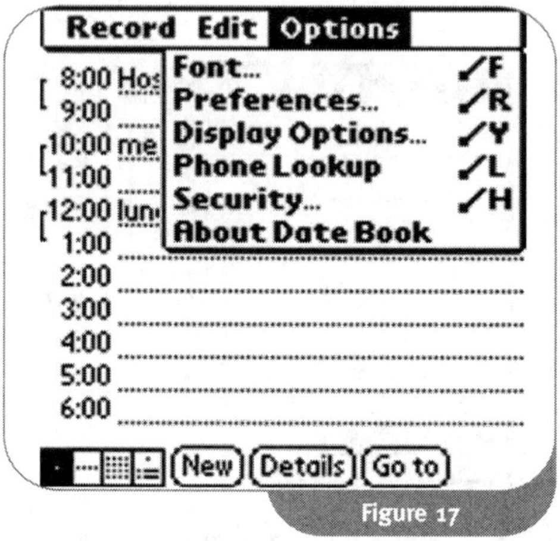

Figure 17

Here is just one of the many neat features. Let's say that we've just made the lunch entry for Bob Marshall (or you can go back to it, tap on it, and the cursor will be placed on the entry). Under the "Options" heading, select "Phone Lookup." Now, if you have previously made an Address Book entry for Bob Marshall, your PDA will magically insert Bob's phone number right here in your Date Book entry (Figure 18).

Another important feature is the ability to set alarms associated with your Date Book entries. You can access this feature by tapping on "Details" at the bottom of the screen. If you don't want to miss an

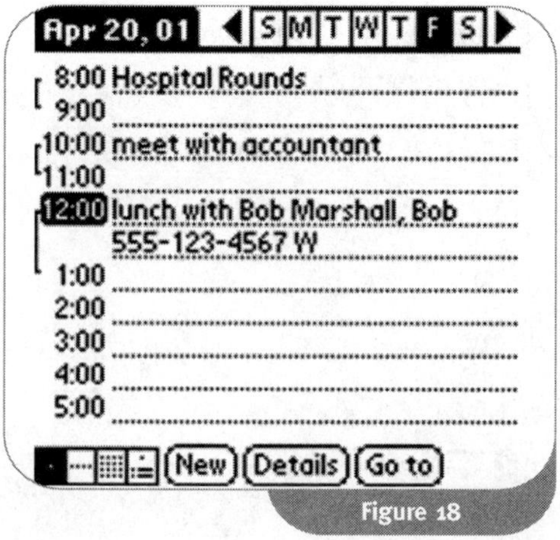

Figure 18

important meeting with the accountant, set an alarm to remind yourself. With your stylus, tap anywhere in the 10:00 entry to place the cursor there. Then tap "Details" to reveal the following "Event Details" screen (Figure 19).

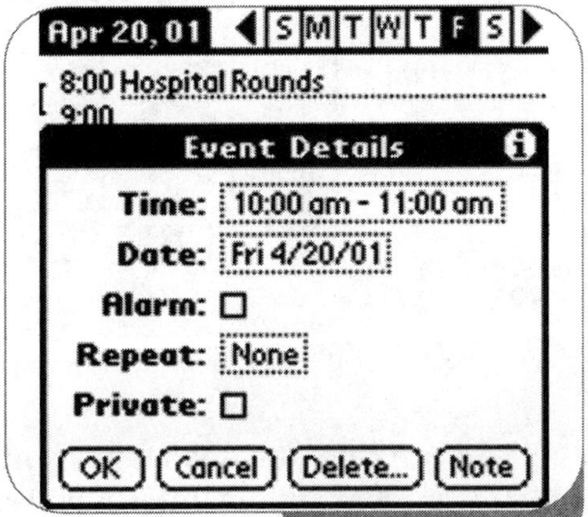

Figure 19

Here we can set an alarm to remind us of our appointment with the accountant. Just check the "Alarm" box to see the choices for how many minutes before the appointment you want the alarm to go off (or hours or days.) After making the selection, tap OK to return to the day view. Here's another tip about your alarms. From the day view screen, tap the Menu button to reveal the dropdown options as we did previously. Select "Options," and then under Options, select "Preferences" (Figure 20).

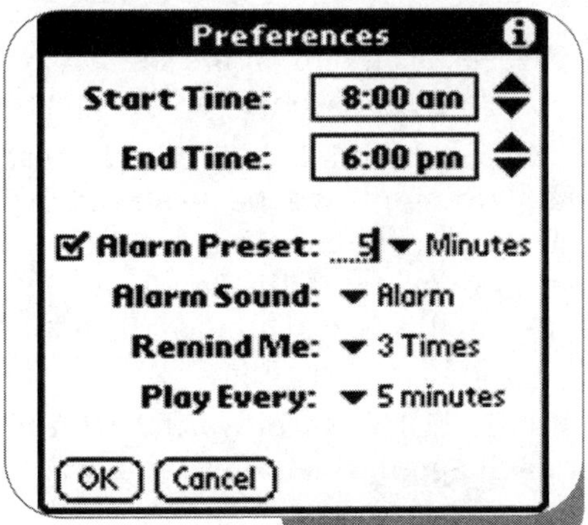
Preferences
Start Time: 8:00 am
End Time: 6:00 pm
Alarm Preset: 5 Minutes
Alarm Sound: Alarm
Remind Me: 3 Times
Play Every: 5 minutes
OK
Cancel
Figure 20

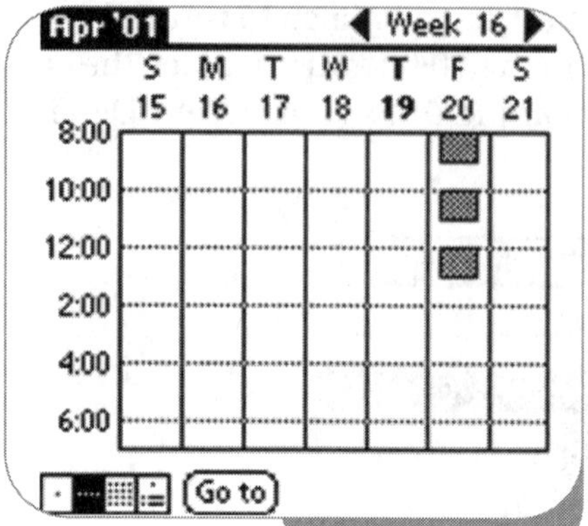

Figure 21

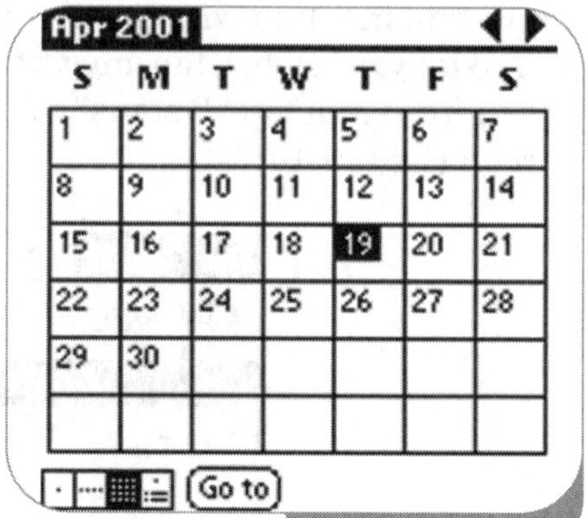

Figure 22

With this screen, you can select which alarm your device will use, how often it will sound, and how many times it will repeat. Tap OK to finish the entry. Now, amazingly, your PDA will remind you of this event even when it is turned off.

Briefly, let's look at the other views available in Date Book: the Week, Month, and List views. Figure 21 shows the Week view for the week that includes the entries we made above for the 20th. Note that bars are displayed corresponding to appointments and their respective lengths. This view provides a quick at-a-glance method of determining when you have openings in your schedule. You can tap on a specific bar to get the details of that appointment to pop into view. Alternatively, you can tap on the number 20 or the "F" to go quickly to that specific Day View.

The Month View works pretty much the same way. You can tap on the next symbol at the bottom of the screen to go there (Figure 22).

The current day will be highlighted (19 in this case), and, again, bars representing appointments will be displayed in their respective places. Go forward or back one month at a time with the arrows at the top of the screen. Tap on a specific date to go directly to the Day View for that date. Tap on the next symbol at the bottom of the screen to go to the last view, the List View (Figure 23).

This figure shows the List View for April 20th. You can see that it gives the entry for each appointment for the day as well as reminds

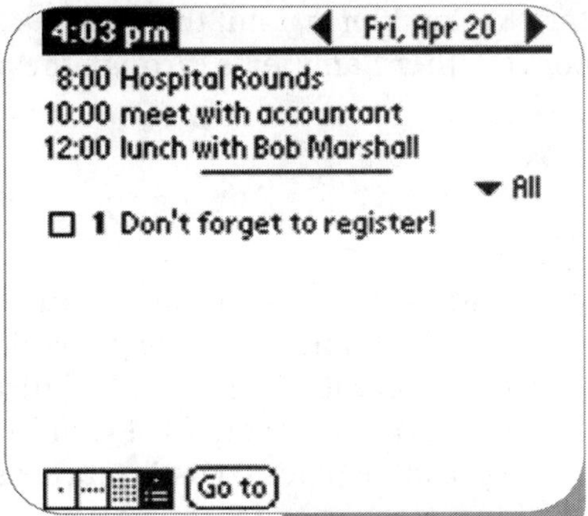
4:03 pm
Fri, Apr 20
8:00 Hospital Rounds
10:00 meet with accountant
12:00 lunch with Bob Marshall
All
1 Don't forget to register!
Go to

Figure 23

the user of items from the To Do list (in this case, the sample To Do item that was installed on my PDA during the setup HotSync). I especially like to search the list view when I know that I've made a particular entry but can't remember the date. When did I have lunch with Bob Marshall? To find out quickly, I simply scroll through the List View.

From any of the Date Book views, select the "Go to" button at the bottom of the screen to go rapidly to another date, month, or even year. These four views and their features constitute the basic Date Book feature. It is rich in features within itself, and you should spend a little time experimenting with the various features, alarms, etc. I think that you, too, will find the Date Book a most useful tool.

Although not all brands of handhelds have Date Book+, it should also be mentioned. HandSprings come with the option of using Date Book or Date Book+. This has additional features, such as the ability to select the opening view for your device, which Date Book+ views are accessed by button pushes, and more alarm sounds and options. More importantly, Date Book+ adds two more views to the standard four: an annotated week view and a year-at-a-glance view, although the latter is tiny and not terribly useful. I like Date Book+'s extended List View, wherein an entire screen of individual entries is displayed. This makes scrolling through a multitude of entries an even more rapid exercise than it was previously in Date Book. Date Book+

may be proprietary to HandSpring, but the features are undoubtedly available to owners of other handhelds through the addition of third-party software.

Memo Pad

Memo Pad is one of your PDA's more intuitive features and one of the most useful. If you're in the habit of writing yourself notes, then you already know how frustrating it is when you've misplaced a note or two. With a PDA, your worries are over. All of your little (or big) notes to yourself are in one portable place. What's more, as with the rest of the four basic functions, you can synchronize your Memos with your desktop PC.

Let's press the Memo Pad button and explore this essential feature (Figure 24).

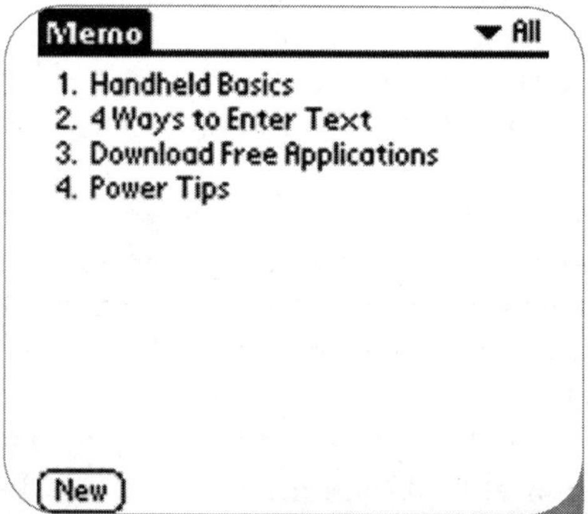

Figure 24

Exactly what you see when the Memo Pad opens depends on how many memos you have saved. Here we see a screen that is something like your PDA will have after first installing your OS. The manufacturer has included four memos for you to read. Note the "All" in the upper left-hand corner. We are currently looking at memos in All categories, although we could quickly and easily assign any given memo to a specific category. You can create new categories, too, by using the dropdown arrow and selecting "Edit Categories." For example, you might want to create different Memo categories for Hospital and Office or a different category for different members of your staff. As with your Address Book, the categories are often used as a convenient means of separating personal interests from business and professional interests.

Later you can see the opening screen of a New memo. The cursor at the beginning of the first line is flashing to let you know that this is where your copy would begin. Because it is flashing, it is your sign to use Graffiti in the Graffiti area to write your memo or to activate the popup keyboard option. It also shows you that this new memo is memo 5 (that is, you have four previously saved memos) and that this memo currently is in the "Unfiled" category (Figure 25). Tap on the "Unfiled" box to select a different category or to create a new one. Then enter your memo. You recall any specific memo by simply tapping on its title. If you want to delete a memo after you are through reading it, just tap the "Details" at the bottom of the screen for that particular memo and select "Delete" from the new popup menu that appears.

To Do List

The fourth basic function is the To Do List. Like the Memo Pad mentioned previously, it is a fairly intuitive function. Press the To Do List button (the one with the checklist icon) (Figure 26).

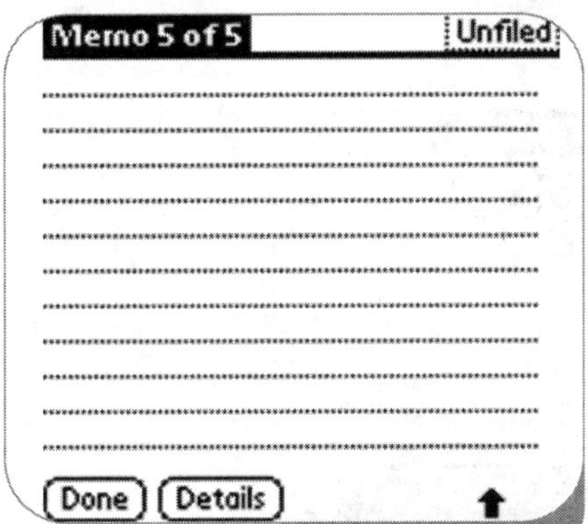

Figure 25

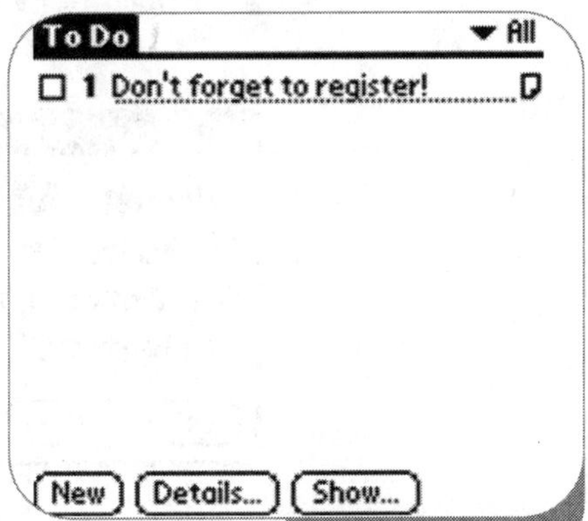

Figure 26

Once more, this is a To Do item that the manufacturer has included in the startup software to show you an example. You can see that there is a small checkbox to the left of the item. You can use this to check off that the item has been completed. In addition, you will see a small icon to the right of the item that indicates that this item has a note attached to it. You can simply tap the note icon to reveal the note or select "Note" from the "Details" view shown in Figure 27.

You can see that this view allows you to give this To Do item a Priority, a Category, and a Due Date, as well as a Note. You can also designate whether you want this particular item to be privately listed. If you opt for privacy, you will be directed to the security application for more detailed instructions about how to hide or mask entries and/or make them available only with a password. The To Do List is a convenient reminder system and a great way to prioritize and get things done.

Other Basic Functions

Calculator/Advanced Calculator. There are a few functions beyond the basic four that are still quite essential. You can tell that these are not as universally basic because they are not assigned "hard" buttons in

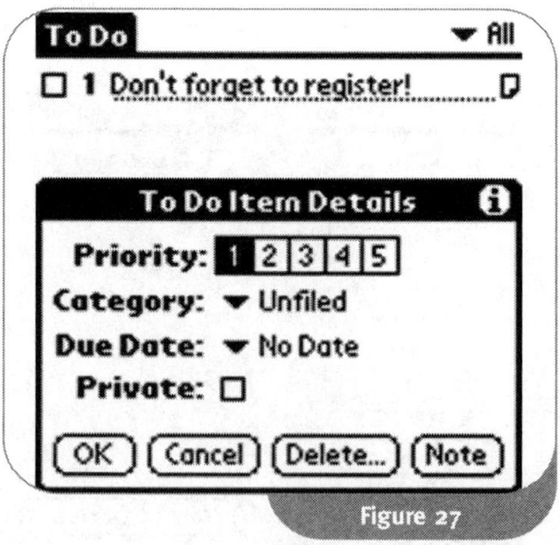

Figure 27

the default settings that come from the factory; however, for some people, one or more of these "other" functions may be more often useful than the basic four. If that is the case for you, remember that you can always reassign a function(s) to one of the buttons; this is done in the Preferences application, Buttons dropdown menu. For now, let's discuss the calculator. Tap on the Calculator icon with your stylus to reveal the screen (Figure 28).

This is handy! No more fumbling for pencil and paper or a separate calculator, as you have one right in your handheld computer. Personally, I think that for medical professionals the calculator function should have been elevated to the significance of a "hard" button. Nonetheless, it's there in the form of a "silkscreen" or "soft" button that you tap with your stylus. This makes sense, too, when you figure that you might want to glance at a Date Book entry, a Memo, or a To Do List. Chances are, however, you won't just be glancing at your Calculator. You'll immediately want to begin calculating something. For this, you'll want to start right off with the stylus, so you might as well have it in hand from the beginning.

Another feature that deserves mention here is the Advanced Calculator function that comes built in to HandSpring products. In medicine, we often need a more advanced calculator function. For example, you might want to convert pounds to kilograms or centimeters to inches more easily. The advanced calculator enables you to do this

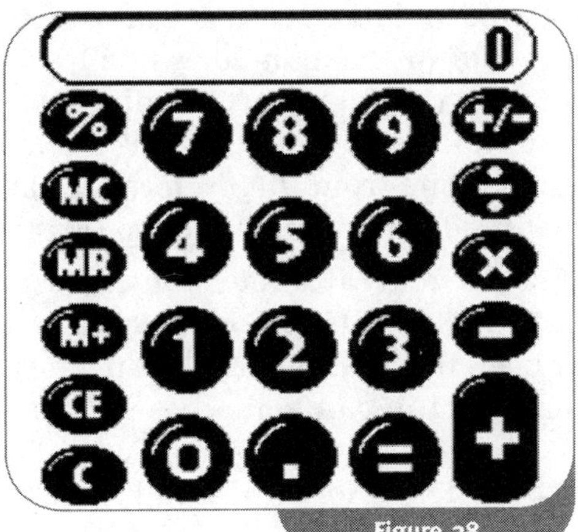

Figure 28

quite rapidly. I was proudly showing a class of physician assistant students the third-party software advanced calculator that I had found (later in the software section) when one of my students astutely pointed out something that I had completely missed. HandSpring models have a great advanced calculator function already built in. You just have to know where to find it and select the right option. Turn on your HandSpring device and tap the calculator icon. Then with the calculator turned on, tap the Menu icon (lower left-hand corner silkscreen button). Three menu items appear at the top of the screen: Edit, Program, and Options. Select Options and then select "Change Mode." Finally, select Advanced instead of the Basic choice. Tap "OK." You should now see displayed a sophisticated advanced calculator. Medical people might then gravitate to "Weight/Tmp," "Length," "Area," or "Volume" options, but "Finance," "Math," and other options are available as well.

Beaming. The infrared "Beaming" feature is another function of your handheld computer that is essential for many people. Although beaming is not assigned a button of its own, you will immediately begin to see its usefulness. Beaming is used by a number of other functions and by a number of third-party software applications as well. In the end, you may wonder how you ever survived without this useful function.

All current PDAs come with the beaming function built in. Depending on your brand and model, the infrared beaming port may be on the side or the top of your handheld. A small red-covered window is both the sending and receiving port for infrared beams. This operates much like your television remote control, but in this case, it's a two-way communication. From the Preferences application, select General from the dropdown menu at the top (Figures 29A and 29B).

At the bottom of the general screen you can see "Beam Receive" with the choice of "On" or "Off." In order to receive infrared beaming from another user, this must be turned on. I just keep mine on so that I'm always ready. You can actually save battery power if you keep this turned off except for when you need it. Personally, I would rather save the frustration of forgetting and just charge my batteries more frequently.

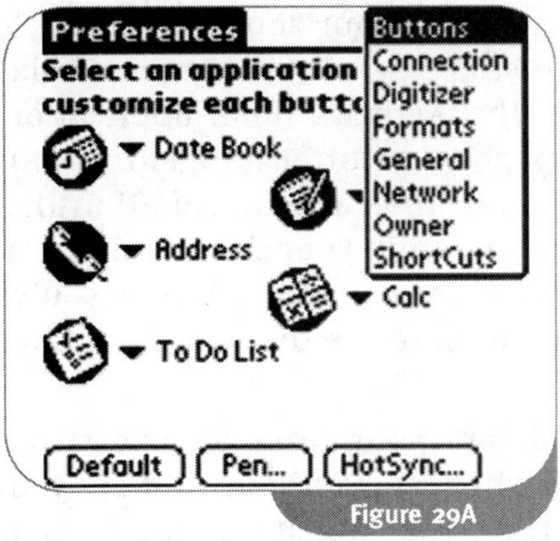

Figure 29A

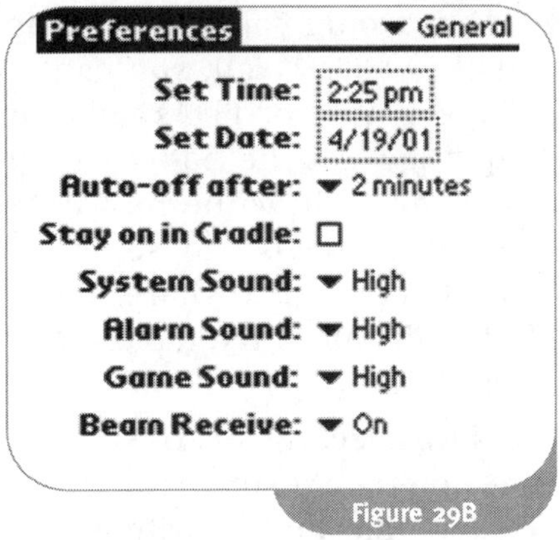

Figure 29B

What would you or another handheld user want to beam each other anyway? First, it can save each of you a lot of duplicated effort. You can beam or receive information from any one of the four basic functions. You can share an address, a Date Book event, a memo, or a To Do List item. From any one of these individual items, tap the Menu silkscreen button. In each case, the menu bar at the top will be displayed, and the first menu item (the farthest left choice) will be "Record." In each case, one of the options for the individual record will be to Beam it ("Beam Address," "Beam Event," "Beam Memo," or "Beam Item"). Tap the Beam choice to begin beaming the information to your recipient by infrared. You do need a line of sight between your respective devices and can only be a few inches to a few feet away. It's not a flawless feature, but when it works it's a thing of beauty and a real time saver. Be sure that the recipient has the "Beam Receive" turned to "On" as described previously. The beaming feature works regardless of brand, as long as the operating system is the same. In other words, you can successfully beam information from your Sony to my Palm because both use the Palm OS. Depending on the individual software involved, it may not be possible to beam between operating systems. In other words, I probably would be unable to beam some things from my HandSpring to your iPac Pocket PC. Feel free to try beaming, even between incompatible devices, as trying causes no harm. Either it works or it doesn't.

How would you like to be able to beam your "business card" to another user? Well, you can quite simply, and it's a great display of the power of PDAs. Just open the Address Book application. Tap "New" at the bottom of the page to begin a new entry. This time, you will *be* the new entry. Enter all of the information that you want to give to somebody else (omit your home phone if you don't want to share it with business contacts). When you've finished your entry, tap the Menu button to see the Record options (Figure 30).

Now select "Select Business Card," and your designated entry will become your business card to beam whenever you want to share your contact information with another user. You can, at that time, select "Beam Business Card" from the same Record screen or simply hold down the Address button for a few seconds until the beaming function begins. This feature seldom fails to amaze new users. Beaming information is fast and accurate. As I have said previously here, when it works, it's a thing of beauty. When it fails to work, it usually means the other user did not have Beam Receive on, the devices were not aligned properly, the distance was too great between the devices, or bright sunlight interfered. Practice a few times with other users to get the hang of it.

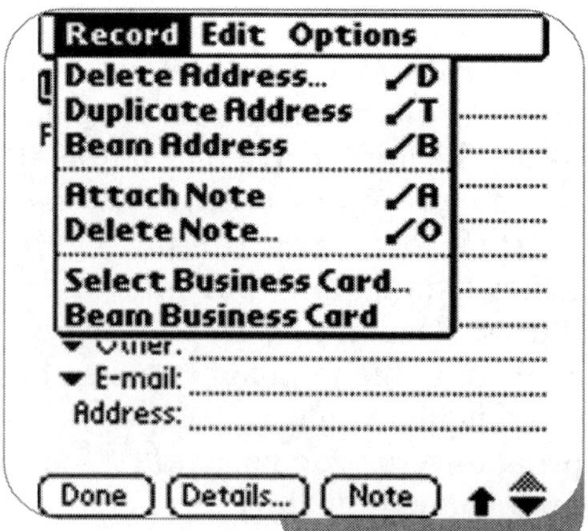

Figure 30

More practicality of the beaming feature will be revealed when we look at other software later; at that time, you'll see how the beam feature will be used to beam information directly to a printer and how you can use third-party software to beam large amounts of patient data to a colleague as you are coming "off service" or when the other user is taking call for you. Handier is hard to imagine.

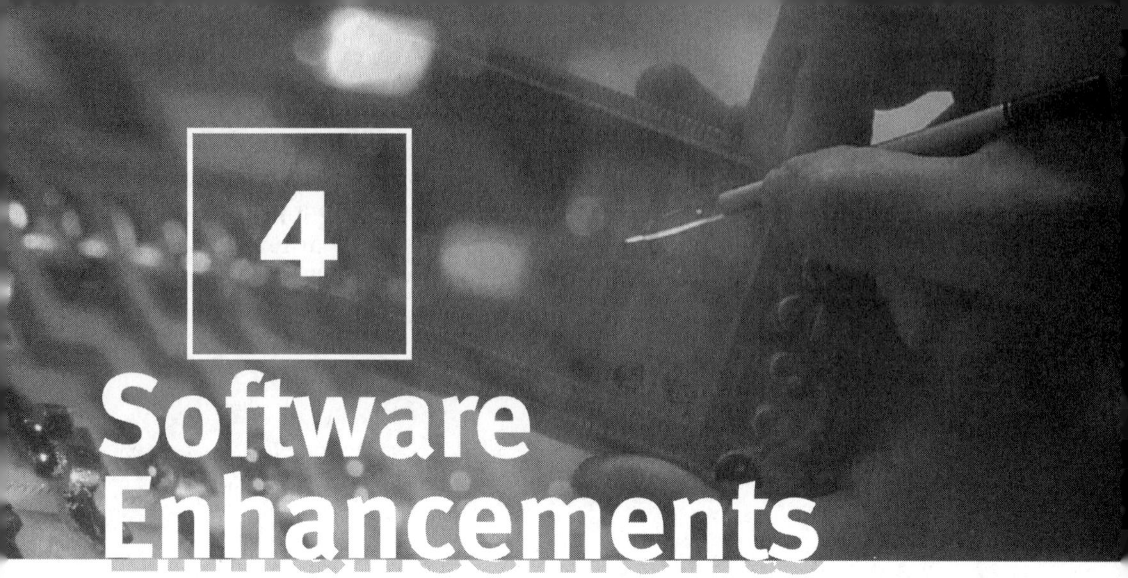

4 Software Enhancements

In this section, we are going to go beyond the basic handheld functions and explore making PDAs more powerful and useful with the addition of add-on software. Some of the add-ons are free if you look for them. Although others cost money, they might be worth the expense. Although this section is not specifically geared toward medicine, you will likely see the medical applicability. In a later section, we specifically explore medical software add-ons.

No handheld is likely to come equipped with all of the software that an individual user might wish that it had. For that matter, two different users will likely have very different ideas about which software should ideally be installed on their respective devices. In addition, licensing issues would undoubtedly increase the cost of a handheld if it included more software. That being said, more handhelds are coming to the market with more software "bundled" with the purchase (much as we have seen in the PC market). There are also issues of memory. The more software that is installed on my handheld, the less memory I have available for other things. For these varied reasons, software becomes a very personal issue. Here we explore some good reasons to look beyond your original software.

Buying and Installing from Disk

Sometimes you might want to purchase PDA software on a disk (usually CD-ROM) and install it directly from the disk source. If you installed on your PC the setup disk that came with your PDA, then you already know how this process works. Basically, you simply insert the disk in your computer's disk drive and follow the installation instructions. The process is much the same for new software that you might purchase for your handheld. Open the disk on your desktop. It will guide you through installation instructions. You will want to save the installation to a folder on your computer where you will save all of your handheld programs. Often the file will come with a Read Me document that will give you further instructions. Then there will be one or more Palm files to install. You will soon learn to recognize the familiar red and green icons (a small green PDA screen with a red arrow swooping into it), which means that these are Palm OS files. Having installed the original setup disk to your PC, these Palm OS files now do a rather clever thing: All that you do is double click on them, and they move directly to your Palm Install file from where they will automatically install to your PDA with your next HotSync. Although Palm files do not open on your PC, your PC recognizes them and performs this maneuver with the help of the Palm software that you first installed.

There are circumstances in which you might purchase PDA software on disk rather than downloading it from the Internet. For example, you might do this if you saw a program that you needed at a local retail store or ordered disks to be sent to you physically. Additionally, some PDAs are now coming equipped with optional software "bundled" by the manufacturer onto the installation CD-ROM. Select which programs you want to add to your handheld, and install them from this setup disk. This is a great way to own software and to maintain a physical backup of the software at the same time. Frankly, downloading software directly from the Internet via your PC and then uploading it to your PDA by using HotSync is more common and perhaps even more convenient in many ways.

Going Online for Software Downloads

The easiest way to search for, review, sample, and buy software for your PDA is online over the Internet. Multitudes of sites exist that feature software for handheld computers. Some are devoted specifically to handhelds. Some sites include handheld sections on their more diverse web sites. Other sites are even more specialized, featuring, for example, only medical handheld applications. Later here, we look more specifically at particular sites that have been very useful. For now, let's just look at the basics of online software.

For the most part it's pretty simple. Go online to the web site, and find a particular software title that you'd like to try. Download it to your PC, and double click on the software application that is now stored on your PC, where it goes to your Palm Install file and is installed to your PDA the next time you HotSync. If you installed the Palm OS software to your PC, then you are set up for HotSync. If you can HotSync, then you can HotSync from any download. The only difference here is that your download is coming from the Internet. The fun is in surfing the available sites for any software that sounds interesting or useful. It is possible to spend many hours with this endeavor. My wife has given up and gone to bed on more than one occasion as I've continued to explore the many software possibilities. I encourage you to explore for yourself, too. I hope that this book will help to make your searches more productive, although there's certainly nothing wrong with surfing simply for fun.

Try Before You Buy

Caveat Emptor—let the buyer beware—is still the universal precaution. However, my new advice is to try before you buy, and the online software offerings usually make this quite easy. I can't think of a single software title that I've seen that does not allow some sort of trial. This may be a limited time trial that automatically expires if the software is not purchased. On the other hand, the trial might be the unlimited use of a "demo" version of the software that is more limited in scope than the purchased version. The trial version might incorporate some other device to convince you to plunk down your hard-earned money. At any rate, it behooves you to give PDA software a good trial. After all, without actually trying it out for yourself, what do you have to go on other than a descriptive advertisement or the advice of another user? How can you predict whether a given software application will fit your needs until you actually try it? Therefore, try before you buy.

Freeware/Shareware/Commercial Software

Software for your handheld computer generally comes in three varieties: freeware, shareware, and commercial software. Freeware, as its name implies, is offered by the software developer for general use without payment or expectation of a fee. Perhaps the developer is just a "nice guy" or is just thankful for the feedback from users in order to create a better more marketable software application down the road. Shareware is readily available software that is shared with other users. The author of shareware usually asks that you pay a voluntary fee. Let your conscience be your guide. Paying the fee (often $5 to $20) usually nets extra benefits, such as free upgrades, no delays at startup, or eliminating pesky reminders that you haven't yet registered the software. Commercial software, as its name implies, is a for-profit venture. Often, though, commercial software is some of the best for its intended purpose. The commercialism underwrites the cost of development.

Basic Software

- Readers: CSpotRun, TealDoc, iSilo, PalmReader, Acrobat Reader, MobiBook, etc.

Different features and different proponents of each reader exist, but it is certain that if you want to get the most out of your PDA, you'll need to install some sort of document reader software. Documents (doc files) abound, short or long, free or commercial, whimsical or informative, but they generally require some sort of third-party translator in the form of document reader software. These, too, can be free or commercial. What you must ultimately decide is whether to part with money for good features in your doc reader or whether the free software will do the job. Again, try before you buy.

The principal free offering in the doc reader category is CSpotRun (by Bill Clagett, e-mail at bill@32768.com). CSpotRun is nifty software. What it lacks in sophistication, it compensates for with its freeware designation. Figure 31 shows the application opened to the beginning of a document file.

You can see that this particular document is the Herbal Reference Guide. Select other doc files by tapping the dropdown arrow next to "Doc." You can also see that the user has several different display type styles to choose from as well as the spacing between lines. The "%" dropdown arrow allows the user to skip, for example, to 50% down into the document. This avoids lengthy scrolling through the document. That's nearly all of the features. CSpotRun is fairly elegant in

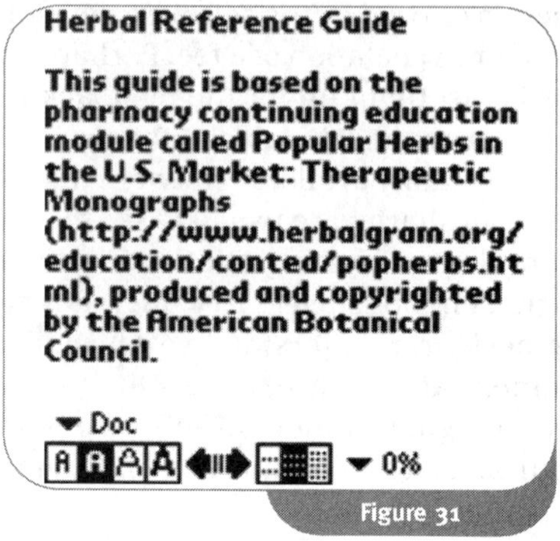

Figure 31

its simplicity. I feel that it definitely deserves a good trial before you decide whether you need something more sophisticated. Who knows, CSpotRun may suit your needs.

One of my favorite commercial alternatives in the document reader category is TealDoc, by TealPoint Software (www.tealpoint.com). Figure 32 shows the same opening screen of the same document, but this time in TealDoc.

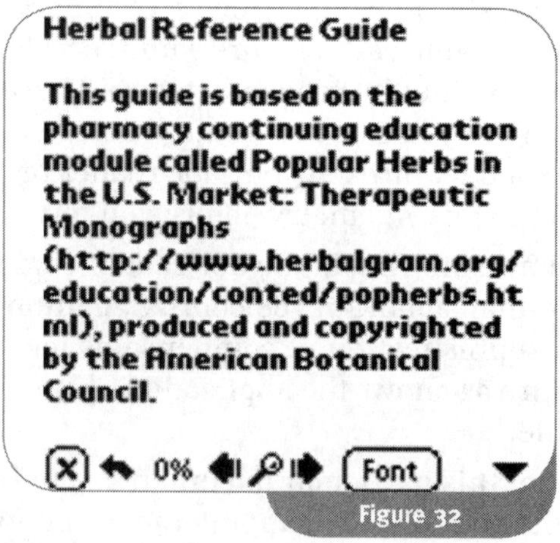

Figure 32

Notice that you still have the ability to select different type fonts or skip to a certain percentage down into the document. The "X" allows you to exit the current document to enter another (e.g., the dropdown arrow in CSpotRun). New, however, are two wonderfully useful features: a little magnifying glass icon that signifies a search capability and the far-right dropdown arrow that allows the user to set and retrieve bookmarks. When navigating a large document, these two features can be as good as gold. TealDoc has several other features as well, but we do not discuss them here.

Another perennial favorite in the category is iSilo, which comes in the full shareware version and in an unregistered free version. Both versions are available from www.isilo.com. Figure 33 shows the same opening screen shot, but with the iSilo free version.

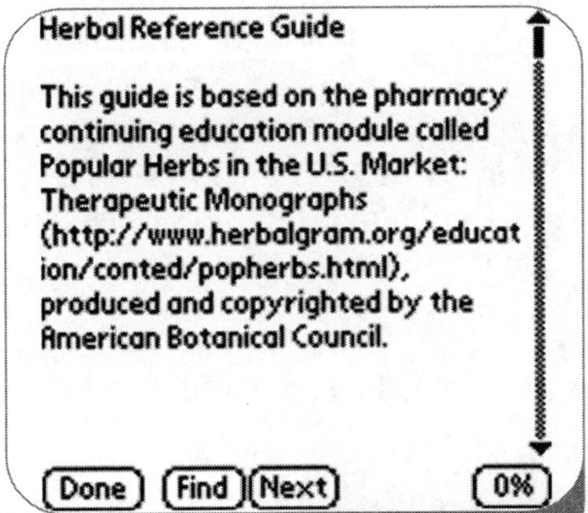

Figure 33

"Done" gets the user out of the current document to the document list. "Find" and "Next" indicate the search function. There's the familiar skip-to-% of document, and the type fonts are selectable but require a couple of taps of the menu button. What's new is the optional scrollbar, shown on the right in Figure 33. This can be another speedy way to breeze through to a particular place in a document. Bookmarks are available in iSilo, too, but again, they require a couple of taps of the menu button. The shareware version of iSilo adds more bells and whistles with the ability to incorporate tables, pictures, and more. It is rich software with a lot of capabilities. The freeware version of iSilo has fewer features, but after all, it is free.

Other worthy contenders exist for the role of document reader on your handheld. I've listed most of them at the top of this section. It would be redundant to go into the features of each of these applications, as they all have a lot in common. They are each, in their own right, worthy of a trial period of use. Decide which features you like best and compare them for ease of use and on a cost basis. You may also find that over time you may want to create your own documents on your PC to transfer over to your handheld. For this, you may need one of the doc readers' desktop versions. iSiloX is one of these. Adobe Acrobat and MobiBook seem to be more visually faithful to the original documents' sources. They are also larger, take up more room, and are more complicated. On the plus side, they are both freeware. PalmReader is another excellent freeware reader. It is necessary for opening and reading certain kinds of documents that I have come across lately that will not open with other readers. Generally speaking, commercial products in the category are more feature rich and undergo more frequent upgrades because they are advanced by profits. I've also found that I tend to carry more than one of these software applications on my handheld because none of them seem to do the entire job for me and because some doc files are specific to different doc readers. I long for a single solution, but have not yet found it.

Databases: HanDbase, MobileDB, Jfile, etc.

Databases comprise another must-have software category for your PDA. Just as I have more than one document reader solution, I find that I need more than one database. Actually, I think that any of the database programs listed previously here (and there are undoubtedly others, too) would probably do the job nicely on their own. Database programs enable a wide variety of applets to be run from them. The problem is that developers write different applets to run with a specific database program. The database programs are not interchangeable in that respect. Software developers, tinkerers, and aficionados of each of the database programs abound. You can see later when we look at web sites that many free or shareware applets are offered and that they usually say whether they run with HanDbase, MobileDB, or Jfile. As with document readers, each of these programs has different but similar features. They are all commercial software, enable you to author your own applets, and generally offer some sort of desktop options as well.

It's hard to describe what database programs do because such a wide variety exists in the applets available and written for them. We'll see specific examples later, especially in the medical software area.

For now, let's just say that database programs are enablers of lists and list reading. You can see later here some of the specific applets written for various database programs and some of their features. Another thing that we do is explore some of the web sites that offer software. Among these are the commercial sites themselves (e.g., www.ddhsoftware.com, the makers of HanDbase) that usually devote entire sections to applets written specifically for their database software. Other sites are not specific to a certain branded database but tell you the database with which their individual applets will work.

Sometimes a PDA user will beam an interesting or useful applet to another user who is then mysteriously unable to open the applet. Invariably, this is because the recipient did not have the proper database program installed on his or her handheld in order to use the applet. For example, I might beam you Alticopeia, the alternative medicine pharmacopoeia. This would frustrate you, and you would wonder whether you had even gotten the program at all if you didn't already have HanDbase installed on your PDA. Alticopeia, you see, will not work without HanDbase. You can acquire them in either order, by the way. Your handheld device will store that Alticopeia applet until such a time as you install HanDbase and enable it.

Image Viewers: FireViewer, etc.

Just as a document reader is necessary for your PDA to read doc files, you need an image viewer to see pictures or drawings on your handheld. Pictures for your PDA are not nearly as ubiquitous as documents, so you may not find this feature as useful as a document reader. On the other hand, few software add-ons are as instantly impressive as a good image viewer for showing off your PDA. I suspect that if I had a color screen model, I'd be showing off more pictures.

FireViewer has become one of the standards in the area of image viewing on handheld computers. Figure 34A shows the PDA desktop with the FireViewer icon. Tap on it to go to the opening screen of FireViewer.

As you can see from these screen shots (Figures 34B and C), FireViewer is shareware that incorporates one of the common shareware "nags." It reminds you that you have not yet registered and paid for the title by "nagging" you with a 10-second delay every time you open the application. Once you get past that, the image table of contents is revealed (Figure 35).

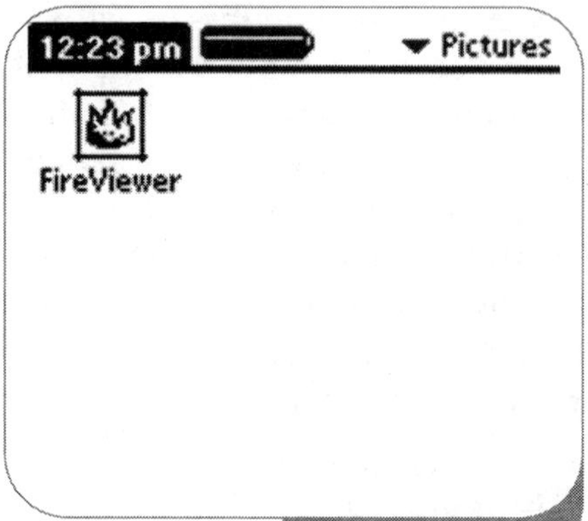

Figure 34A

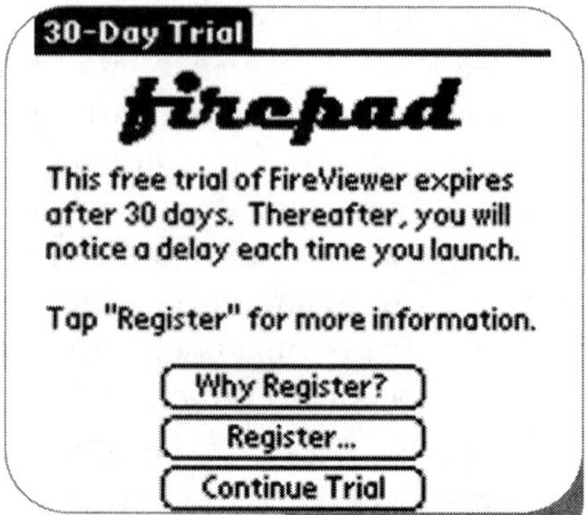

Figure 34B

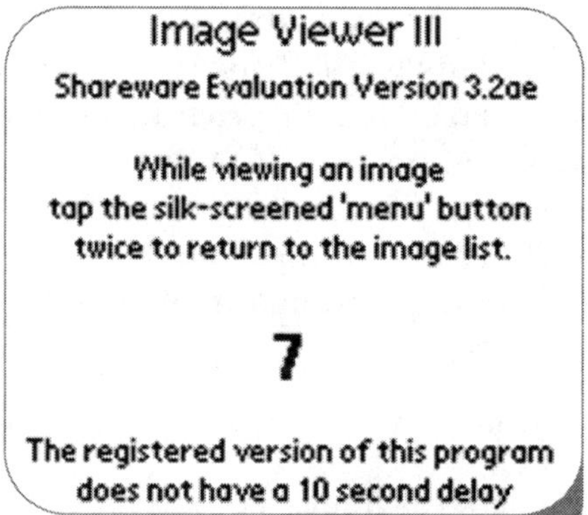

Figure 34C

You can see from this table of contents that I have already installed several images: Some are family pictures, and others are anatomical drawings. You can see that the sizes of the images are included to the right (in pixels × pixels) and that there are several features in a control bar at the bottom of the page (Figure 36).

After tapping on "Skull (Front)" in the table of contents, I come to the screen shown in Figure 37.

Here you can see the full-version frontal view of the skull with labels attached. Notice that the left icon in the tool bar is highlighted, indicating that this is the full-image view. A neat feature in the full-image view is that you can move the image around on the screen with your stylus to have a better view of different parts of the image. Tap on the various tool bar icons for other functions,

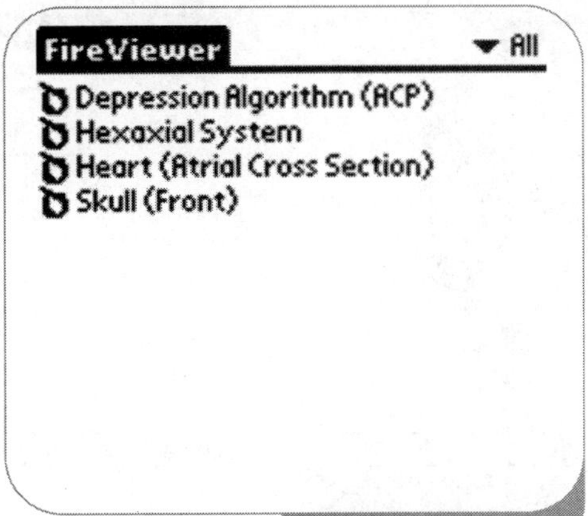

Figure 35

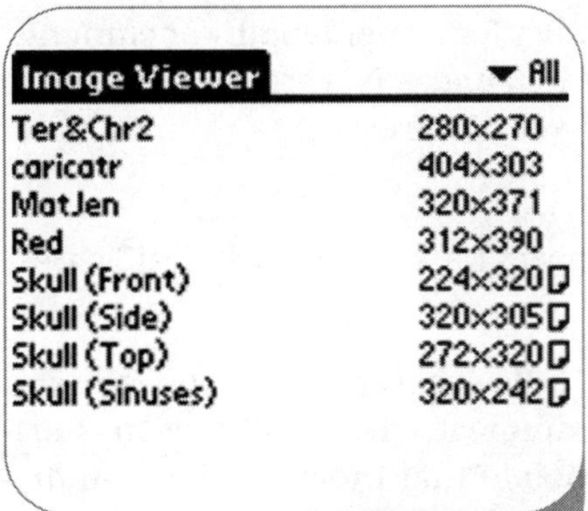

Figure 36

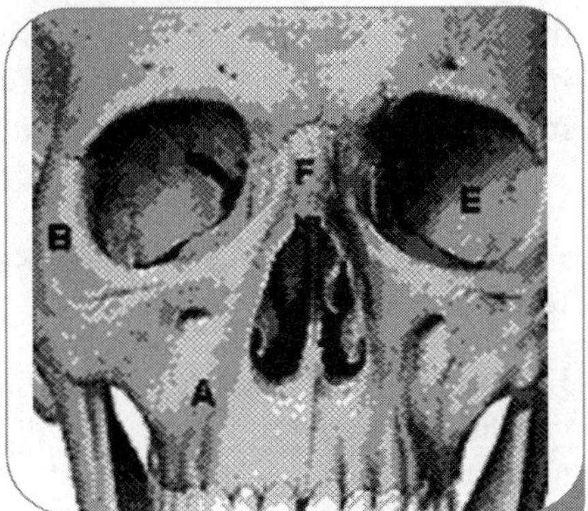

Figure 37

such as viewing the image in a smaller version, beaming the image to another user, adding notes, or viewing the notes that go with the attached labels (Figures 38A and B).

Where do these images come from? The anatomical drawings (e.g., skull) have been posted on the Internet as freeware. However, I said that I had loaded family photos into FireViewer as well. A very versatile feature of most of the image viewers is that they also have a desktop image converter available. With this feature, you can convert electronic images (as from a digital camera) on your PC to images that can be HotSynced to your PDA. It's all very exciting. One caveat is that images on your PDA are memory hogs. Compared with docu-

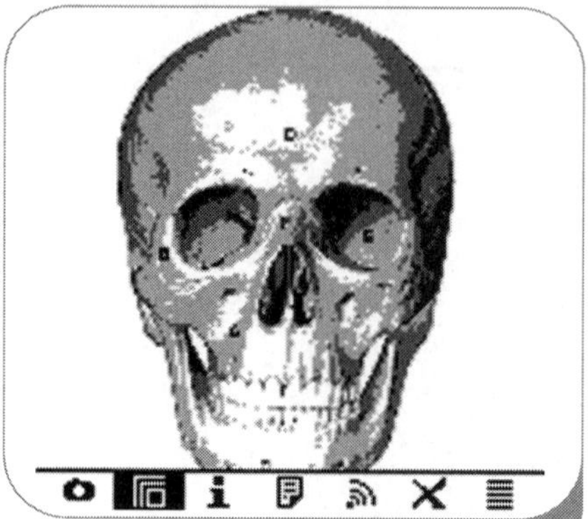

Figure 38A

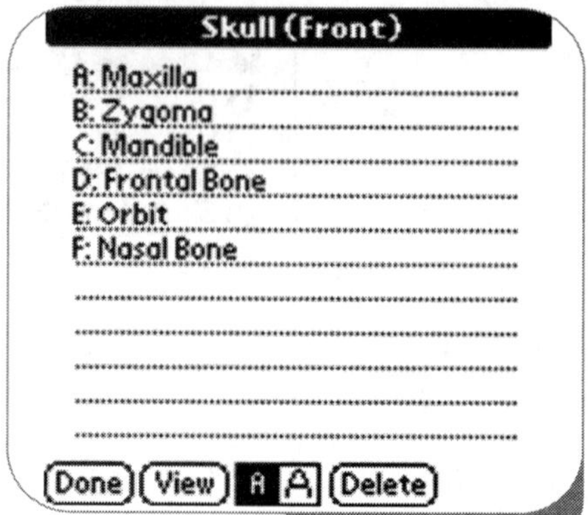

Figure 38B

ments, which take up very little memory for rather lengthy documents, images take up a lot of memory for each image. Nevertheless, the right images can be very instructive and very impressive.

■ Hacks: HackMaster, TealMaster, Keyboard Hack, Clock Hack, TealGlance, TealEcho, TealLens, etc.

Hacks, I am told, are file extensions, little programs that squeeze extra versatility from your standard PDA applications. It's all very mysterious to me, but you'll quickly appreciate that there are a few indispensable hacks. The good news is that they take up very little memory. The bad news is that if you install enough of them to your handheld computer, hacks seem to have an annoying tendency to cause your device to crash. It's generally not a crucial matter, but it is definitely scary and a time waster. My advice is to try a few different hacks, one at a time. If you notice an increased tendency to crash, you could eliminate the last new hack installed to see whether that clears up the problem. Nevertheless, hacks are still worth having and using, albeit in small numbers. In order to use any hacks at all, you need to install one of the hack-enabling programs. Again, these are small programs themselves that allow you to manage your hack programs and turn them on and off according to your needs. Several of these hack-enabling programs exist. The HackMaster icon is shown in Figure 39. Click on it to open HackMaster.

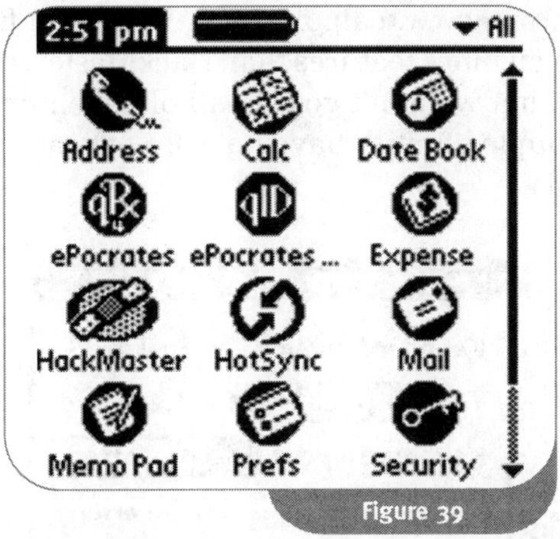

Figure 39

Once HackMaster has been opened, you have the option of "turning on" any of the hacks that you have installed on your PDA. As shown here, only two hacks have been installed (discussed later). You can see a checkbox to the left of a given hack that you would select to turn on this particular hack. The "+" sign to the right of a hack opens up an option screen for that hack, whereas the "?" displays copyright and ordering information for the hack. You do not have to remove or uninstall a given hack to disable it. Simply deselect the hack by unchecking the box to the left of it (Figure 40).

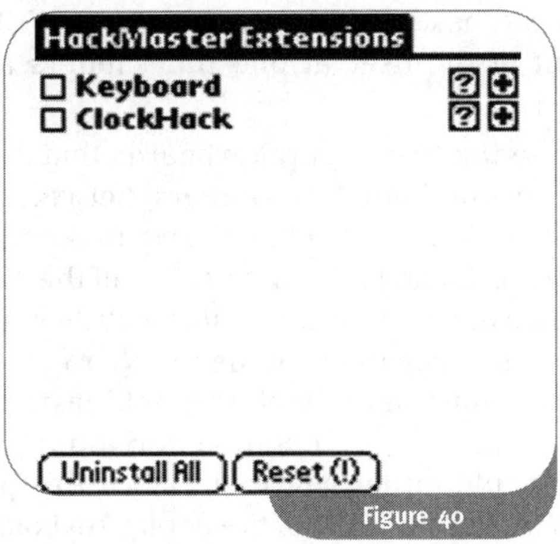

Figure 40

TealMaster (from www.tealpoint.com) is another fine hack-enabler program with even more features than HackMaster. It deserves a careful comparison, but we don't go into all of its features here. Instead, let's look at a couple of must-have hacks: Keyboard Hack and Clock-Hack (Figure 41).

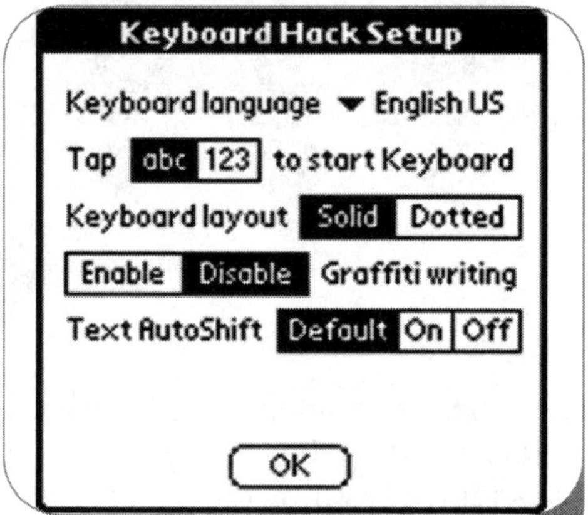

Figure 41

Here you can see that we've tapped on the "+" to the right of Keyboard to select the options for this hack. If we tap on the two highlighted areas (abc and Solid), this is what we'll get the next time we're in a program and want to use the popup keyboard to make an entry (as in Address Book, Date Book, Memo Pad, or To Do List). For me, this is the best. The entire familiar QWERTY keyboard is laid out in front of the user at one time, letters and numbers together (Figure 42).

Contrast this to the two popup keyboards that are built into your PDA, one for letters and one for numbers, between which you must typically bounce back and forth in order to make the simplest entry. The Keyboard Hack doesn't eliminate either of the old possibilities either because you can now tap on the little numbers in the lower right corner of the Graffiti area to bring the number keypad up just as before. In addition, you can go back to HackMaster and disable the Keyboard Hack at any time. Of course, for you this may seem nonsensical as you would rather be (or already are) a proficient Graffiti user. Nevertheless, I'm still a fan of the popup keyboard and thus enjoy this hack (Figures 43A and B).

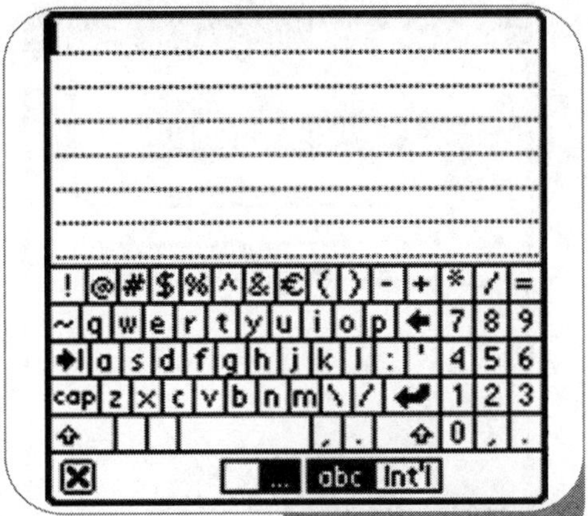

Figure 42

Another hack that seems handy is the ClockHack. Here you can see the ClockHack preferences that were accessed by tapping on the "+" to the right of the hack. Selecting the highlighted preferences shown will place a small digital clock in the bottom right corner of your PDA screen in most any application. This is handy; however, if it becomes annoying or gets in the way, you can always disable the hack by deselecting it (Figure 44).

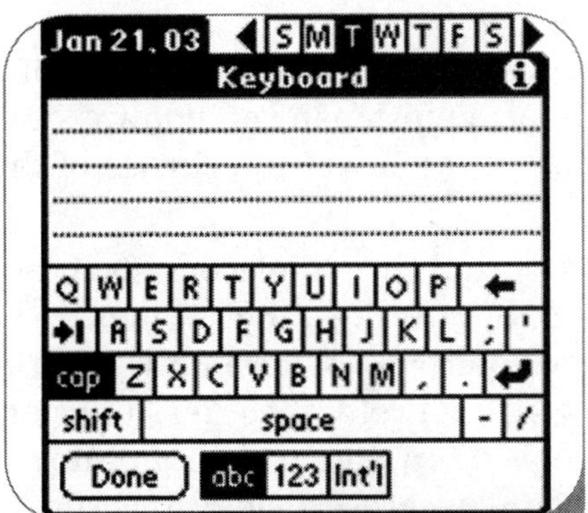

Figure 43A

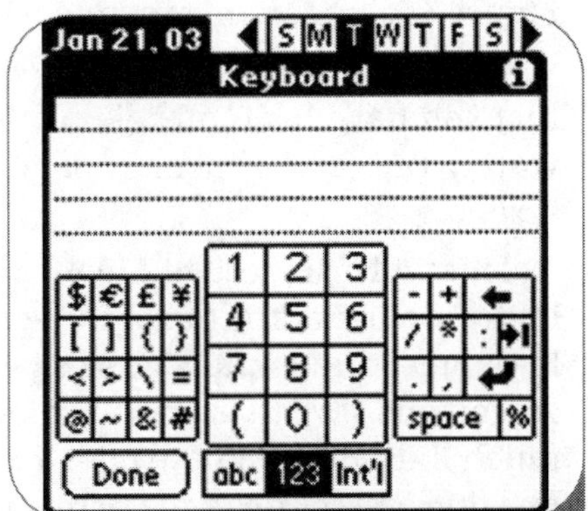

Figure 43B

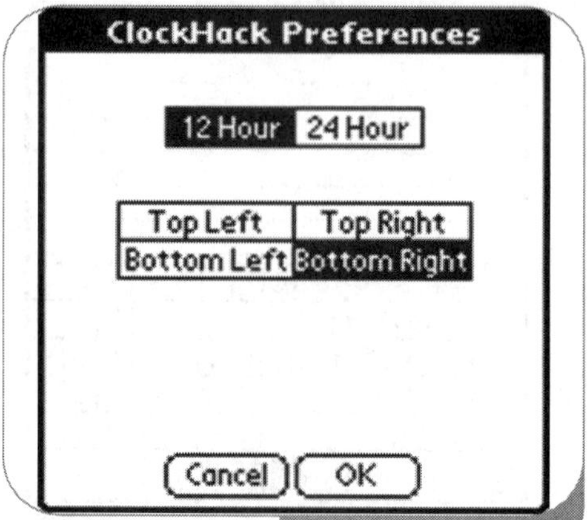

Figure 44

HandWrite, PicChat, Scribble, etc.

For some handheld users, this category is the handiest and the most fun. I would loosely categorize these applications as graphics programs, although that's a bit misleading. These applications are small yet powerful additions to your PDA. If you're a veteran note taker and note keeper, then you'll appreciate these programs. In fact, Sony must have deduced the nearly universal appeal of this type of program because it has included the full-featured Clie Memo on its latest models. For the owners of other models, the first of the add-on graphics programs is HandWrite, which is a great freeware application (by Hiroki Urushibata, e-mail at uruki@mail.wbs.jp). Its icon is shown in Figure 45. Tap on that to enter the program.

You will come to the screen shot shown in Figure 46 and imagine that you have been mistakenly teleported to Japan somehow. Not to worry. Tap on the turning page icon in the lower left corner of the screen.

This will bring you to a blank page with various tool icons displayed in the toolbar at the top of the screen. HandWrite allows you to scribble notes, draw maps, or sketch body parts anywhere on your PDA screen and save these masterpieces for later reference. Yes, it's pretty much like your old note pad. The tools allow you to choose different line thicknesses for your writing instrument, erase, delete, time stamp,

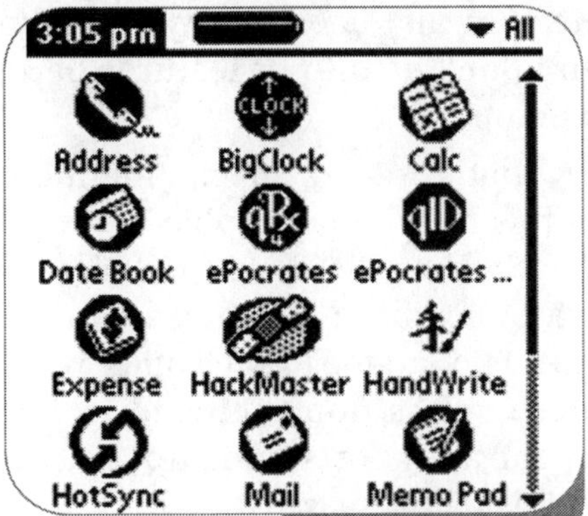

Figure 45

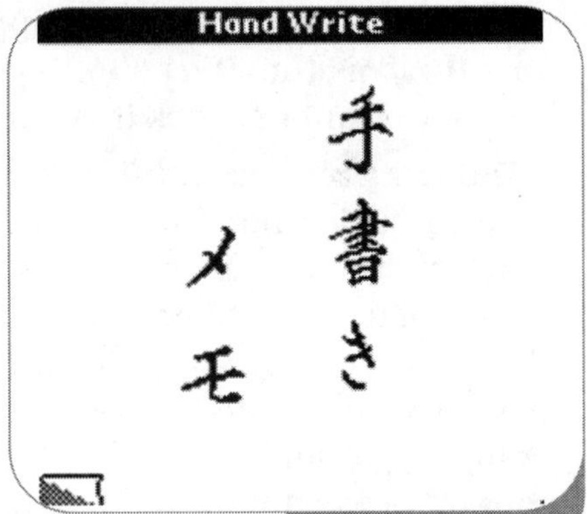

Figure 46

or turn the page to the next memo. Importantly, this is not character recognition software (i.e., it doesn't take your scrawlings and convert them to letters or words) (Figure 47). However, what HandWrite does, it does brilliantly. After all, why should you have to carry around pencil and paper when you have your trusty PDA by your side?

Clie Memo works pretty much the same as HandWrite, having essentially the same controls. With the color models, you even have the ability to select the color of your pen from among black, blue, or red. You can vary these and the pen width within the same note page for some very diverse effects.

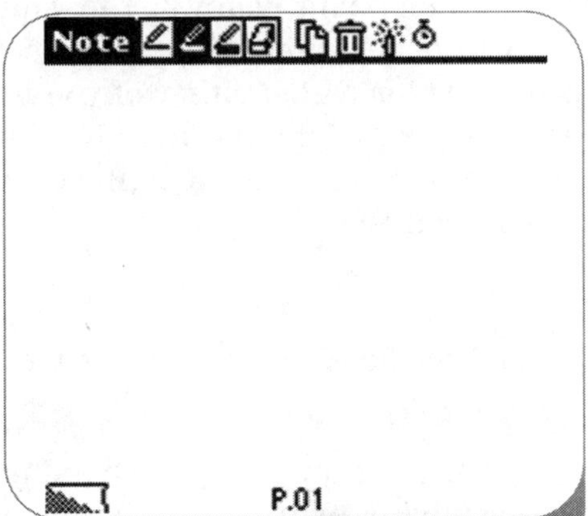

Figure 47

Scribble is another similar application that does pretty much the same thing as HandWrite. Although I don't go into its features here, you might want to check it out and compare.

Another program in this category that deserves special mention, however, is PicChat. This application is truly unbelievable, if somewhat less practical. If two handheld users have PicChat installed, they can scribble notes to each other while beaming in real time to the other user. Imagine scribbling a game of tic-tac-toe to each other without ever getting caught passing notes in class. You get the idea. The two users would have to have their infrared ports lined up, and although the execution isn't flawless, it is truly amazing.

Beam Box, Beam Pro, etc.

Beam Box, Beam Pro, and other similar programs give added versatility when sharing contents and subprograms with other users. You will soon find that you have collected quite a few documents in your document reader, databases in Mobile Database, or applets in HanDbase that you might want to share with a colleague. In many cases you couldn't do that because your PDA's built-in beaming function won't split out the contents so neatly for you to beam individual items. Beam Box and Beam Pro fix that oversight in your handheld's software. You will find that with either program you can beam virtually any of the previously named items. First install Beam Box to your PDA, and then beam Beam Box to your fellow user before you actually try to beam some document. Seemingly, the only exceptions are programs for which either of you has paid licensing fees or which have been copyrighted. These have little "lock" icons next to them and will not beam, even with Beam Box or Beam Pro. Check them out and compare.

Dictionaries: Noah, BDicty, Translate, etc. (regular, thesaurus, foreign language)

Dictionaries and similar programs for your handheld computer are enormously popular, judging by the great variety available. To me, this was a natural growth progression of the PDA. What could be handier than to have a dictionary, a thesaurus, a foreign language translator, or any of a variety of medical dictionaries (just to name a few)? In most cases, simply install the base dictionary program, and then install one or more modules according to your needs. For example, install the freeware Noah (as in Noah Webster) dictionary and then install its content word set (either WordNet Small at 1329K or WordNet Full at 5139K), depending on your needs and memory capabilities. Similarly, you could install either of the fine commercial programs, Beiks BDicty or DDH Software's Translator. Then purchase and install their respective modules according to your needs, your pocketbook, and your PDA's memory capacity. I've used DDH's Translator with the Spanish module for the occasional Spanish-speaking patient or the Italian module for a trip abroad. The translator works in both directions between two languages and can do words and phrases. Dictionaries are almost limitless in their potential and variety. The limit is the amount of memory that you have to devote to them, as most are memory consuming. The trade-off of a smaller dictionary is that the word you're searching for may not be in there.

■ BigClock/StopWatch

At the risk of sounding redundant, the category of timekeepers is one that I have found to be quite useful. The amazing thing to me is that my two favorite programs in this category are freeware: They don't cost a penny!

Let's start with the simplest first. This would be StopWatch (by Jacob Copsey, http://www.copseystrain.com), which has just one simple function, no bells or whistles: It simply acts as a fine graphic stopwatch (Figure 48).

As you can see from this screen shot, Stopwatch is quite basic. Tap in the designated area to start the stopwatch, and tap in the designated area to stop the stopwatch. That's it. The numbers at the top of the screen show the time to the 10th of a second. The stop and start areas of the screen are large enough that, if necessary, (shudder), you could even activate them with your fingertip. I like the no-frills approach of Stopwatch and the fact that it occupies a paltry 9K of your PDA's memory. You can't beat that. Be aware, however, that to conserve battery power, your PDA will likely turn itself off after 2 or 3

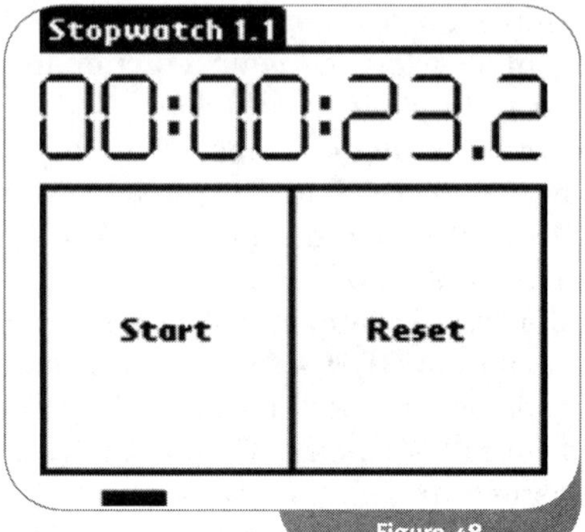

Figure 48

minutes. The Stopwatch will still be running in the background, but you will need to turn your device back on to see it again.

One of my all-time favorites in this or any other category of handheld software is BigClock (by Jens Rupp, e-mail at jens@gacel.de). This one small program (only 34K of memory) has gotten so much attention and use by PDA owners that I'm surprised it hasn't been purchased and bundled with other installed software. Kudos are given to Jens Rupp for creating one of the most useful, elegantly simple, and flawless programs available for the handheld computer thus far. Figure 49 shows the screen shot of the BigClock icon on the PDA desktop. Tap on this to open the program.

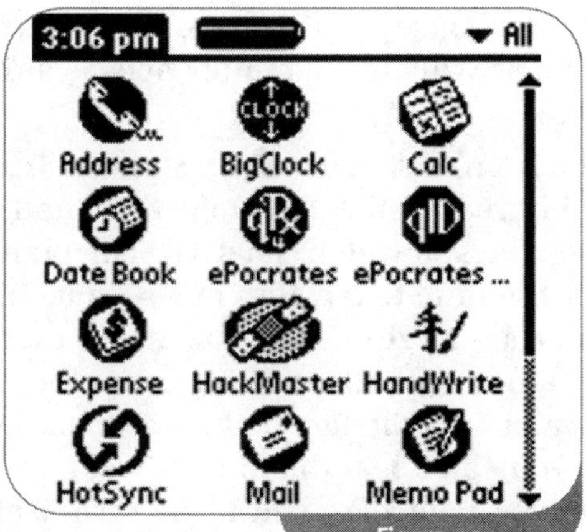

Figure 49

As you can see below, BigClock opens up to . . . well, a big digital clock! Notice in the lower left corner that we are in the basic "time" mode (Figure 50). Day and date are also displayed.

You could also tap Alarm at the bottom of BigClock to access the alarm clock feature. Here you see the alarm clock screen. It shows

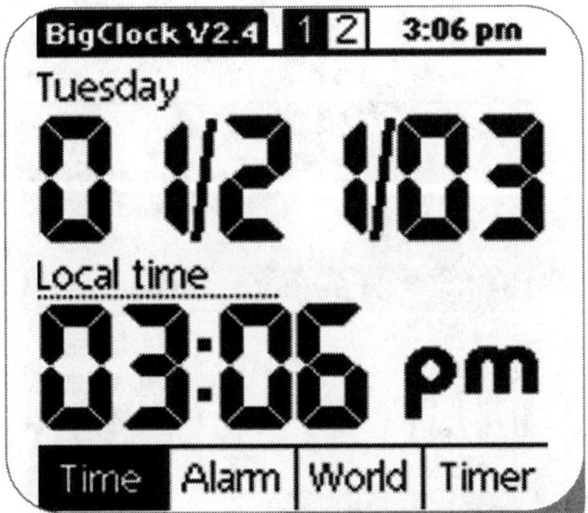

Figure 50

that you have the ability to set two separate alarms, each with one of four different alarm sounds. I use this feature extensively when I travel. I don't even have to request any wake-up calls. Be careful of two things: that you actually turn on the desired alarm by selecting the box to the left of the alarm (neither of the alarms shown has been turned on) and that you make sure to highlight the proper day (Saturday a.m. for alarm 1 and Sunday through Friday a.m. for alarm 2). Amazingly, the alarm clock, just like the rest of BigClock, runs in the background of your PDA. Turn your device off, and the alarm you set will still go off . . . like clockwork (Figure 51).

If you tap on the menu icon (lower left-hand portion of your PDA screen), you will open the following dropdowns: Options, Sounds, and Info. Use these to access and select your various preferences within BigClock (Figure 52).

If you tap on Sounds, you'll see the dropdown menu: Sound 1, Sound 2, Sound 3, and Sound 4 (Figure 53).

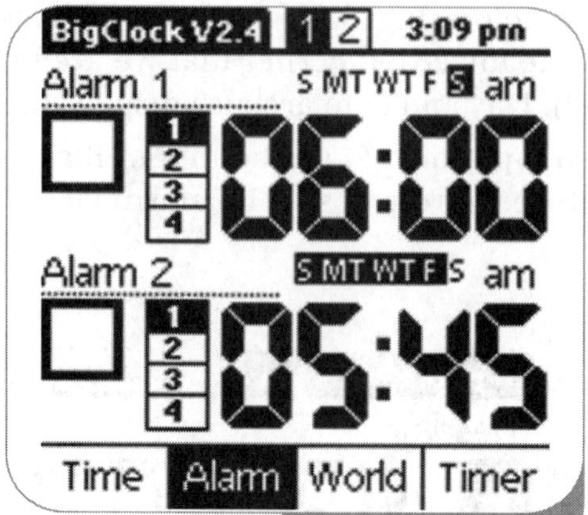

Figure 51

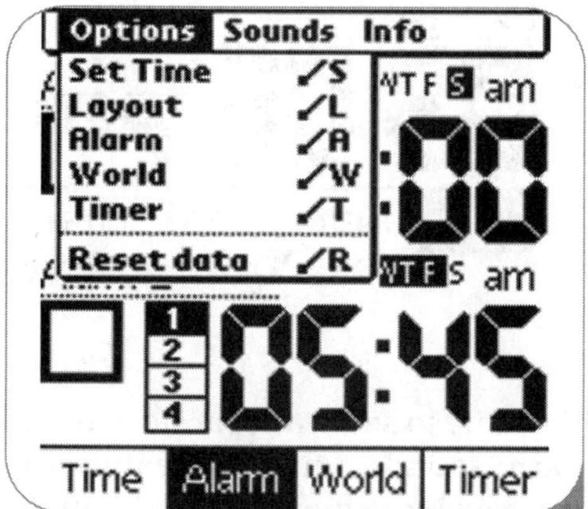

Figure 52

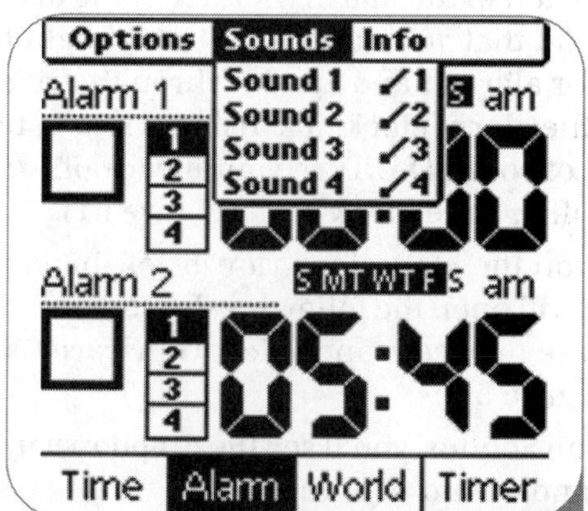

Figure 53

Here we have selected alarm Sound 1 (Figure 54), and you can see that this screen allows the user to test the sound and completely customize it. This is an incredible amount of versatility for such a small program. You may never even want to touch the preset alarm sounds, but isn't it neat to know that you could if you wanted to? I like this feature for showing off my alarm clock to new PDA users. If they don't already have BigClock, they invariably ask me to beam it to them.

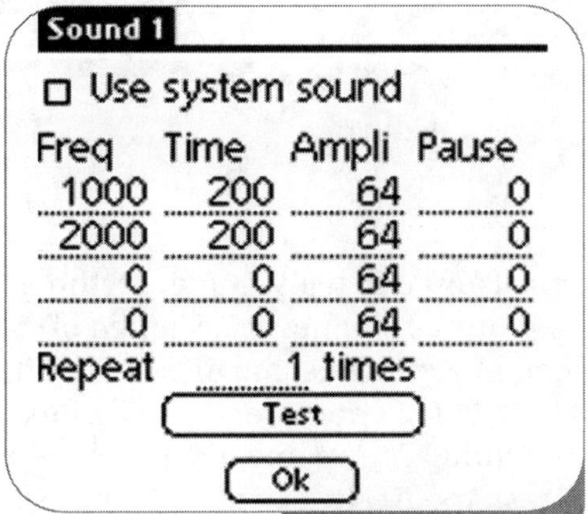

Figure 54

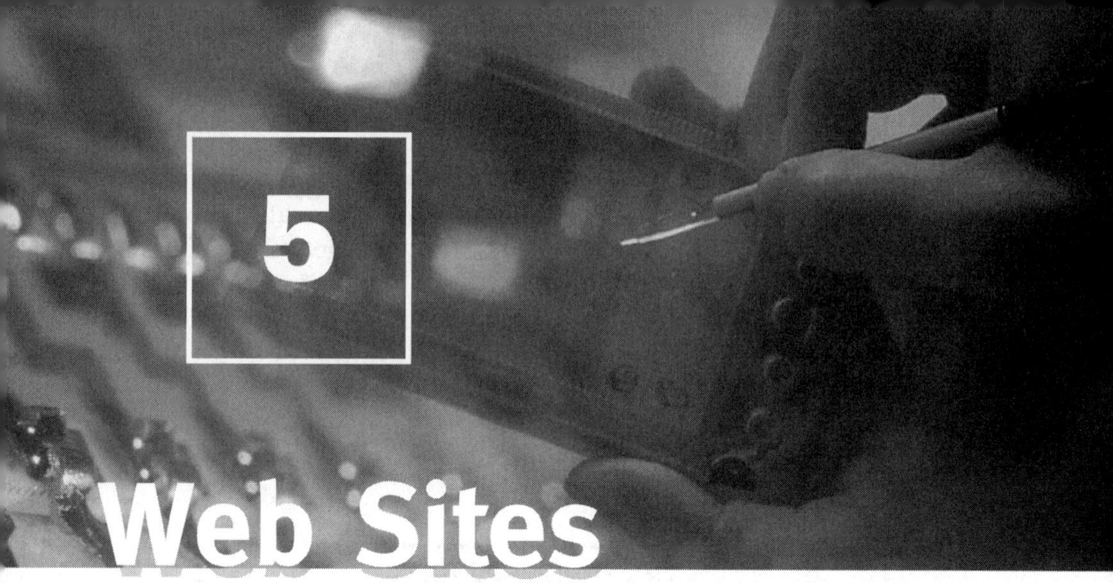

5

Web Sites

Now the fun begins! You can truly find everything you ever thought of (and quite a few things you never dreamed of) for the PDA on the Internet. This section explores some of the web sites that have been most useful to date. This is not intended as an exhaustive compilation. Web sites are fluid: They come and go. Here we divide the sites into general interest, medically oriented, commercial, and miscellaneous. Later we go into specific software.

Generally speaking, I suggest that first timers spend quite a bit of time at a new web site getting used to its features and offerings. You don't do this in a rush, at least not at first. Plan to spend at least half an hour with a new web site. This is not something you do on your way out the door to an appointment, as you might miss some good features. Later, after you've spent some time with a web site, you can check back for brief visits just to find out what's new. Some sites will even put you on an update list, if you sign up, just to notify you of new items that are added to their site. I find this quite handy.

General

General-interest web sites as a group are quite diverse. Here I highlight just a few. Certainly, there are more sites than these, and more will have appeared by the time you read this. However, these have proven quite useful over the past few years.

Zdnet (www.zdnet.com)

ZD stands for Ziff-Davis Publishing, the publishers of PC Magazine (among others). The site is well organized, has a good search feature (try entering the name of a Palm OS or Pocket PC software application that you're looking for), lists most popular downloads, offers commercial products for sale, and more. I recommend spending a great amount of time with this site. If you want to keep even more up to date, subscribe to one or more of their free e-mail newsletters.

Access ZDnet by typing the previously mentioned address into your Internet browser. You will see that the ZDnet site is quite diverse. To access the relevant PDA portion of the site, go to the heading marked "Go Mobile," and click on it. Various categories about handheld computing are available here for exploration, including hardware, review articles, and more. I especially enjoy browsing the "Downloads" section, with particular attention to the Palm OS offerings.

PalmGear (www.palmgear.com)

PalmGear is a very nicely organized web site. As its name implies, it gets right down to the handheld stuff that we're really interested in. An easy-access table of contents of the site is listed on the left side of their web page. Click on "Tips & Tricks" to access hundreds of helpful hints that handheld users have sent in. Click on "Software" to view one of the most complete PDA software listings available on the web. Here you can easily browse the available software by category or by type of application (whether it's a document or a musical program, etc.). There's also a handy search feature at this site. Simply type in the name of the program for which you are looking, and you will likely find it at PalmGear. Check out "Calvin's FAQ" (frequently asked questions), which answers many basics and gives great references to books and magazines devoted to handheld computing. This is a rich site, and I would therefore suggest spending some time browsing and getting to know it. Your time will be well spent.

■ TuCows (www.tucows.com)

Despite the annoying banner advertisements, this is one of the most entertaining PDA sites. TuCows has a lot of downloads, many of them free, and rates them by the unique "cow count" system. Favorite software gets a rating of 5 cows instead of 5 stars. Well organized, this site features many categories of downloads, medical and otherwise. Be sure that you are browsing by Palm OS category, if that's what you're looking for. Besides the cow count rating, this site easily shows whether the selected software is freeware or shareware, how big the file is, and when it was written. These are all useful items to know before you download something to try it out. By clicking on a software title that looks interesting, you get a more detailed description of what the program will actually do.

Again, you can spend many hours browsing this site for its many useful and fun downloads. I think that it's definitely worth checking it out periodically to see what new items have been added. TuCows has even made periodic checks for new software easier by adding the "What's New" section and the "What's New Archive" of previous new entries. If you check the site on a regular basis, then all you have to do is browse the "What's New Archive" since your last visit.

Medical

Some web sites go far beyond the general interest area. Here we explore some of the more useful sites that are specifically geared to the medical PDA user. Once more, this certainly isn't all of the available sites, and new ones are being added all the time.

■ pdaMD (www.pdaMD.com)

This is a great web site for the medical professional (I have written reviews for them). This is a must-read site for anybody who is contemplating the purchase of a handheld computer or anybody who is new to handheld computing. With the site's "Learning Center" feature, you can easily walk through the purchase decision process and solve problems that are common to new users. The tutorials in this section walk you, step-by-step through every process, are easily searchable, and are well laid out.

pdaMD features articles and reviews of software and hardware, which are all amazingly relevant to PDA use in medicine. Thousands of other medical professionals are interested in and are using PDAs every day and are often contributors to these reviews and articles.

You can also access software and hardware in the "Products" section. Here the commercial nature of the pdaMD site is more evident, but it is forthright, too. Products clearly have their price tags and are neatly organized and categorized for browsing. This section makes electronic catalog shopping great.

Another way to surf many of the software offerings of pdaMD is through HealthyPalmPilot (www.healthypalmpilot.com), a sister site to pdaMD. Check out their Healthcare Resource Index, with hundreds of medical software offerings, neatly categorized and labeled as to freeware, shareware, etc.

My favorite part is that you can subscribe (on their home page) to receive pdaMD updates free via e-mail. It's free, and if it becomes too intrusive, you can always cancel it. You can similarly subscribe to free e-mail updates of new listings on HealthyPalmPilot.

HandHeld Med (www.handheldmed.com)

Currently, I don't find the web site for HandHeld Med as full-featured as pdaMD. Nonetheless, it has a lot to offer medical users. You sign up as a user for free, and then access the web site later using your log in. HandHeld Med's commercial nature is clearly evident, but they have many good, classic software offerings available, as well as a free reader that is used to read their e-books. They have partnered with the American Medical Student Association, which is more evidence of the wide acceptance of PDA's among new medical professionals.

ACPonline (www.acponline.org/pda)

This site, I think, epitomizes the medical professionals' PDA site of the future. As handhelds become ubiquitous in medicine, we will see more mainstream medical groups and associations incorporating PDA information into their sites for the benefit of their members. I believe that the American College of Physicians–American Society of Internal Medicine is at the forefront of that movement, and they are the second largest physician group in the United States. This site is the PDA portal of their general web site. The offerings are few for now, but they have quality and are credible. I look forward to more from this site in the future. For now, check out their excellent free documents, including an Ethics Manual and a Bioterrorism decision support tool for medical professionals.

Medical Schools and Medical Student Groups

Still apparently in its infancy, I expect this to become one of the more fruitful areas for medical web site development related to PDAs. More PDAs are being used by more medical students in more medical schools, and the experienced upperclassmen are increasingly having more tips to pass along to their underclassmen. Some of the more savvy schools and users have put their experience on the Internet to share.

If you search the web sites and links of various medical schools, you may find sections or portals devoted to handhelds, PDAs, or Palms. Check them out. I can't offer too many examples in this area for now, as I'm still investigating myself, but one you might want to peruse is the Cornell site (http://class2003.med.cornell.edu/palmpilot/palm.html). Although this hasn't been updated recently, it offers a few pertinent tips for new users with links to some of the sites we've included here. Another fine example in this category is the University of Alberta (Canada) Medical School PDA portal (www.msa.ualberta.ca/computing/handheld/links.html).

EctopicBrain (http://pbrain.hypermart.net/) is a brilliant site that a doctor maintains. It includes handheld basics, links, downloads, and more. Dr. Kent Willyard, author of the site, is quite a software developer in his own rite.

Commercial

Commercial PDA web sites abound. These are the home pages of the software developers and their marketers. How else is one to spread the word? Although they clearly have their own agenda and the name of the game is selling software, they can still be quite informative and up to date. At these sites, you can compare the features and prices of the latest commercial software direct from the manufacturer. You can try out a demo or make a final purchase, all over the Internet.

■ Handango (www.handango.com)

This is definitely a commercial site, as much of what is here is for sale and is not free. However, the site deserves surfing time. A lot of useful information can be found here, as well as some of the best medical software for sale. Although the emphasis may be on medical software, room is still available for general interest software for sale here, too. Some great games and utilities exist for Palm OS as well as links to other sites. Handango, too, has a free newsletter for which you can register.

■ Handmark (www.handmark.com)

Handmark is another commercial PDA web site. It is a slick and well organized site with many appealing software offerings, although you'd be hard pressed to find any medical applications among them. Handmark, however, is the maker of MobileDB (reviewed previously among the database software). MobileDB, as we see later, has many medical applications. Therefore, after all, I would rank this as a quite important web site for our purposes. Besides, Handmark has some neat commercial game offerings for the PDA (e.g., Monopoly and Scrabble). These are unbelievable board games, especially on color handhelds.

■ DDH Software (www.ddhsoftware.com)

DDH Software is another fine commercial software site. The folks at DDH are in the game to sell software; however, if you browse their site, you will find that they have several good medical software offerings. In fact, one section of their site is labeled "Medical Solutions." DDH's main claim to fame is their HanDbase database program. Thus, reminiscent of the Handmark site mentioned previously, you'll find here a "Gallery" of free applets that use HanDbase. These are mostly free, and many of them are good medical applets. We'll explore some of these in particular later.

■ TealPoint Software (www.tealpoint.com)

TealPoint is one of my favorite web sites, despite the fact that it's commercial. For me, the reason is simple: They have some really great software. Most of the offerings here are shareware, and many of them are worth buying. TealDoc is an excellent document reader with good features. TealMaster is a Hack manager, sort of like HackMaster on steroids. TealGlance is a neat application that flashes important reminders from your Date Book or ToDo List each time you turn on your handheld. TealEcho makes your Graffiti strokes show up (as though your stylus had ink in it) to help you master Graffiti faster. TealMagnify lets you enlarge any area of the screen that you tap with your stylus. TealInfo allows you to read special databases called Folios that were written specifically for it. There's more software. The TealPoint folks also have libraries of documents and Folios on their web site. There, too, you can sign up for a free updates newsletter.

Miscellaneous

Some web sites of interest to medical PDA users just don't fit neatly into any one category. At the same time, they're important enough that they deserve mention here.

■ MapQuest (www.mapquest.com)

My wife can affirm that I am one of those alpha males who hate to stop and ask for directions. On the other hand, I know that I'm directionally challenged enough that a good map can be my best friend. If you haven't yet discovered MapQuest on your PC, you're in for a treat. At the MapQuest site, you can print (for free) a detailed street map and/or driving directions between almost any two points in the United States. For me, the really neat benefit is that you can also download the MapQuest software (also free at the web site) onto your PDA. Then when you get driving directions, simply HotSync and have your directions with you at the tap of a stylus. I have found these maps and directions to be accurate and convenient. How did I live without them for so many years?

■ AvantGo (www.avantgo.com)

AvantGo is a unique concept, as you don't need to have a wireless Internet connection to enjoy web content on your PDA. The key is AvantGo's mobile internet service. You sign up for the service for free, while registering for one or more of hundreds of free "channels." You could select news, sports, stock market reports, or entertainment magazines. You name it. Almost all of the familiar favorites are available free at AvantGo, including *The Wall Street Journal*, CNN, *The New York Times*, *USA Today*, *Car and Driver*, *Boating*, and many more. After you pick the channels, the new content is downloaded to your PDA with your next HotSync. You could do this daily if you choose. You can also turn off certain channels, add or subtract channels, or keep the content you already have and do a HotSync without AvantGo. It is a very versatile system. Certainly your downloads are not complete issues of magazines, but the content can be quite informative and entertaining nonetheless.

AvantGo also works quite extensively with business, industry, and institutions to offer mobile solutions to their various needs. They will customize their products or offer you your own channel to which others would then subscribe. This has apparently found wide applicability among sales forces.

AvantGo is handy, but I found that I was taking up a lot of memory with the various magazine downloads. Ultimately, my subscriptions (all free, mind you) have had to give way to other programs on my handheld. If you have room to spare, however, or waiting time that could be spent more profitably, then I recommend that you check out AvantGo.

One of my latest finds on AvantGo is Dr. Rose's Peripheral Brain. I added it to my AvantGo channels to install it to my PDA and then set my HotSync setting for AvantGo to Synchronize. This installed the Peripheral Brain content to my PDA. I then went back to my HotSync settings and set AvantGo to Do Nothing. This way, in future HotSyncs (which I do all the time for various reasons), the Peripheral Brain content will be left alone on my handheld, and no further memory or time will be taken up with AvantGo HotSyncing. Any time I want to upgrade Dr. Rose's Peripheral Brain, I simply reset AvantGo to Synchronize at HotSync.

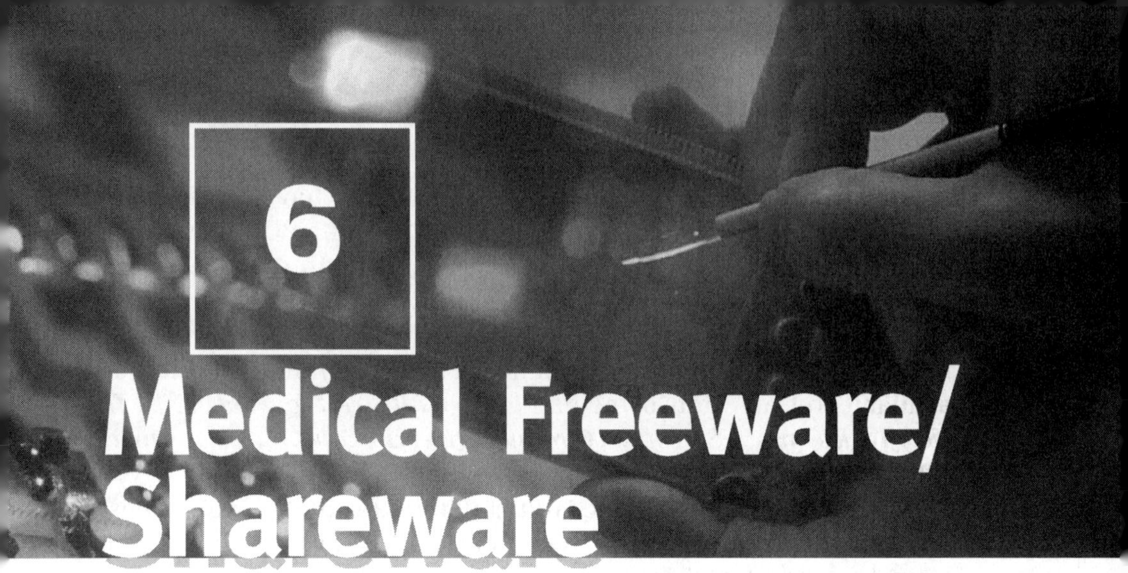

6 Medical Freeware/Shareware

In previous sections, we've looked at typical software enhancements for your handheld, as well as some of the web sites where you might find them. Specifically here we'll explore some of the myriad useful medical shareware and freeware. This category is abundant and expanding rapidly, and thus, this section is likely to be instantly out of date. However, it will be useful to see some of the variety that is available and has been helpful in the past.

Freeware and shareware are interesting from several perspectives. Naturally, we all appreciate such software because of its economy. My advice to students is to find out what freeware or shareware meets your needs before spending limited resources on commercial products. Don't get me wrong. Commercial products certainly have their advantages, and thus we'll explore them in the next section. It's amazing to me, on the other hand, how many good offerings there are for medical professionals in this money-saving category.

So why is there such a vast array of free or low-cost medical products for the PDA? One reason is that these products are sometimes in development. Developers often experiment with a new product, put it out there free, and then improve the product as they receive comments and suggestions. The result is a tried-and-true product that has been field tested and had the wrinkles removed. Now the developer can confidently charge for the product and has a ready demand for it. Another reason for freeware and shareware, apparently, is that some people are just inveterate tinkerers. They just like experimenting. They may come up with a program or applet that fills a need for them and logically conclude that it could be helpful to others. I think that medical professionals often fall into this latter group. You will see quite a few products from the ranks of medical students and doctors. These are savvy people who have embraced handheld technology, applied it to medical problems, and decided to share it with others in the medical field.

Some of the applets and programs that are reviewed here have stood the test of time, continue to be posted to the web, and continue to be useful. A caveat to anybody using freeware/shareware (but especially medical professionals) is to consider the source. Often the source material or even the author is unknown or not easily discovered. Certainly, any clinician would want to use these programs with caution and only to supplement their clinical skill or expertise.

Doc Files

One of the most fruitful areas for medical professionals in this category is document files. I especially like to look for these files at Memoware or TuCows; however, other good sites also exist. You will need one of the document reader programs to open and read these applets. We have discussed both the sites and the document readers previously. Among document files, more than any other category, the size of the file in kilobytes (K) is proportional to the content of the document. Here are some titles that you might find useful:

1. Abbreviations (32K). The practice of medicine uses many abbreviations. This is a handy reference, but the source is unknown.
2. Black Book 2.0 (178K), by Seth D. Scholl, D.O. This is a neat reference for a document file. The author has solved some of the navigation problems inherent in a doc file with the inclusion of both a navigable table of contents and bookmarks, as shown in Figure 55.

   Here we see a section of the navigable table of contents. If we tap on the "A" square, we come to the screen shown in Figure 56.

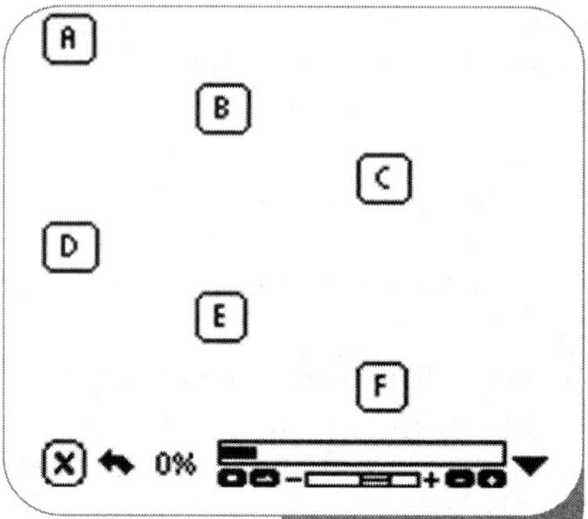

Figure 55

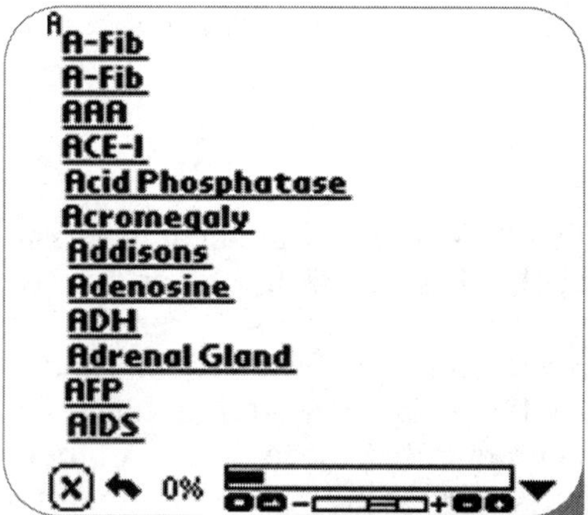

Figure 56

If, in turn, we tap on "Addisons," we come to the entry for Addisons Disease, which looks like Figure 57.

Notice the succinct outline style of entry. The content is brief, but a lot of information is contained in this 178K document. Black Book can be navigated with the use of bookmarks that the author has built into the document. Not all document readers include this feature, but here is a compelling reason for seeking out a reader that does (Figure 58).

Here you can see one of the bookmark pages superimposed over the navigable table of contents. There are 24 bookmarks included in Black Book that can quickly get

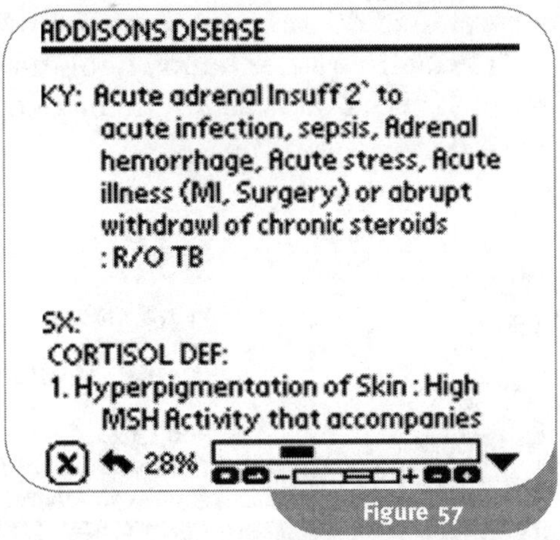

Figure 57

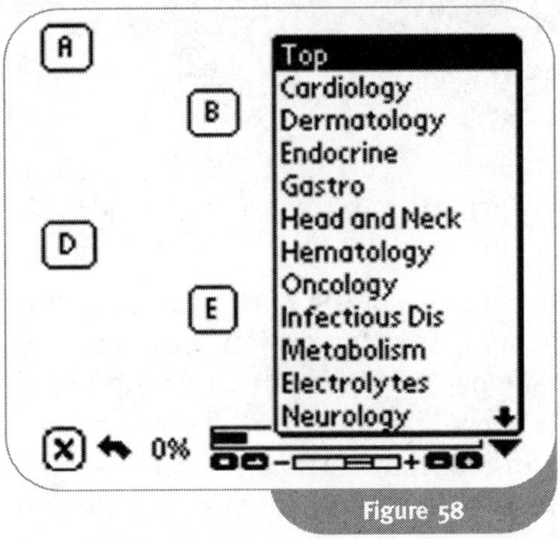

Figure 58

you to the chapter of the document that you want. Once you are there, you may have to do a bit of scrolling to find what you're actually looking for. This is, as I said, a lot of information crammed into one document. It's a bit cryptic for the beginner but is full of useful information for the more experienced clinician. It deserves a look.

3. Chapter 1: Upper Respiratory Infection (3K). Here's a small document that is illustrative of what is available. Although I can't recall where I got it, who authored it, or where the rest of it is, it is nonetheless succinct and useful. The tip-off is the small size of the document. The other clue is the name. I suspect that this is a sample or

demo version of other chapters to follow at a retail price. What's left? Some rather handy bookmarks as you can see here. Next to that is a sample page on Epiglotitis (Figure 59).

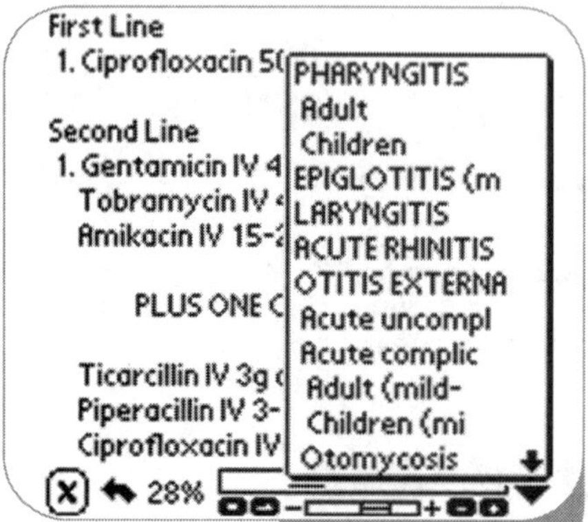

Figure 59A

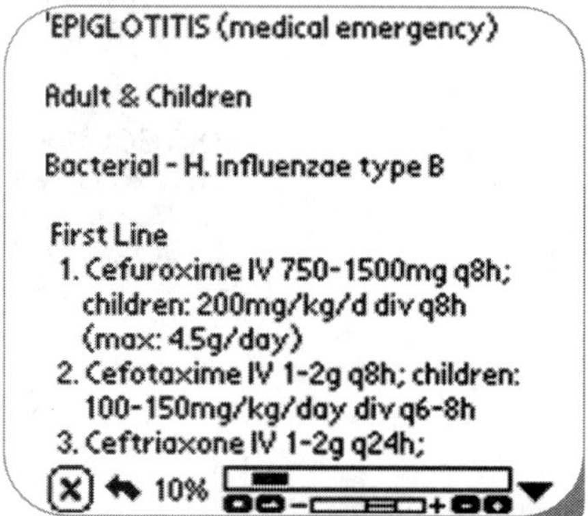

Figure 59B

The information is sparse but useful. The problem here is not knowing the age of the information.

4. Common Herbs (10K). Although the author and date are unknown, the information seems useful and handy. You may see patients periodically who are taking some of these herbal medications. This is good information that is arranged neatly. Here we see a section of the bookmarks highlighting herbal products and the associated piece if one were to tap on the Aloe Vera bookmark (Figure 60).

Farther into the bookmarks is a section about specific complaints. Tap on constipation, for example, and you'll go to suggested herbal remedies for this complaint (Figure 61).

My major complaint about this document is that it just missed going far enough. I would greatly like to have seen suggested dosages. Other than that, I think this is a winner.

5. EKG Reference (3K), compiled by Kent Willyard, M.D. This is a handy reference with key reminders bookmarked conveniently. It even includes a nice graphic of

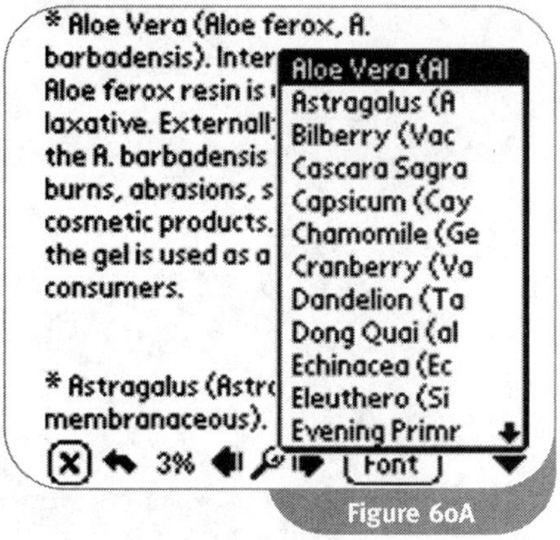

Figure 60A

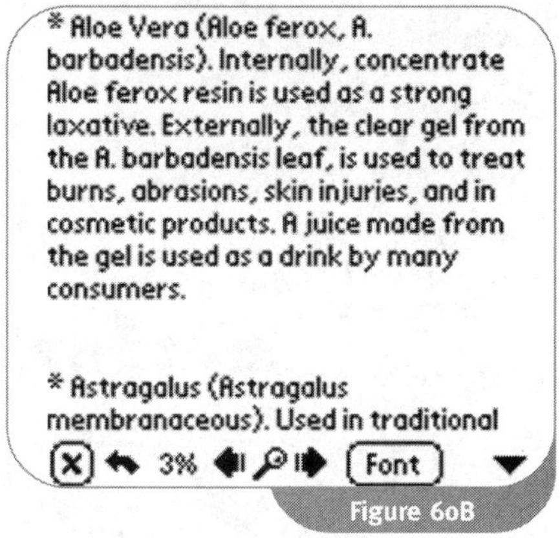

Figure 60B

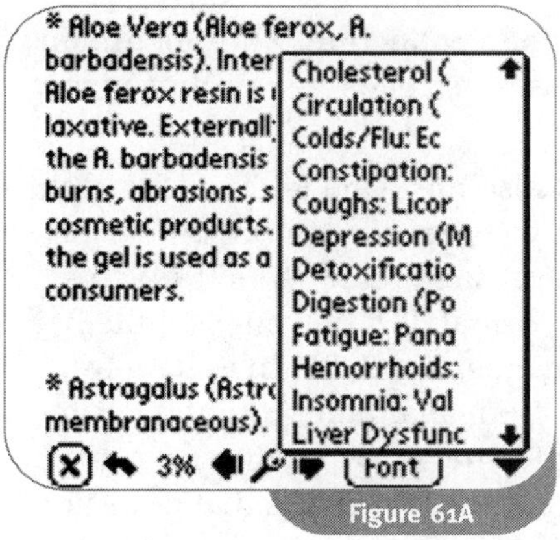

Figure 61A

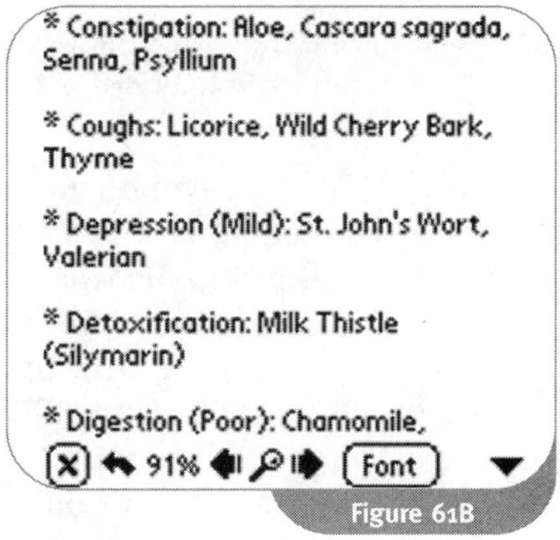

Figure 61B

that pesky hexaxial diagram, which plagued me in physician assistant school (Figure 62).

Look for this author again, as he is a prolific tinkerer and has posted many useful medical titles in various formats. My hat is off to Dr. Willyard, as he enjoys sharing with his colleagues.

6. Eponyms Doc (178K), by Andrew J. Yee, M.D. (http://eponyms.net). Have you noticed how many medical conditions, signs, and other entities are named after specific people? You might take some of them, such as Addison's Disease or Homan's Sign, for granted; however, would you immediately recognize Gaucher's Disease or Klumpke's Palsy, among the hundreds of others? I know I certainly can't make that claim. Dr. Yee comes to the

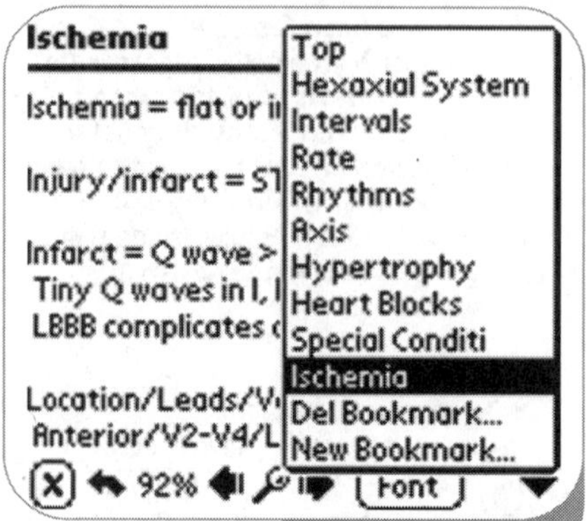

Figure 62A

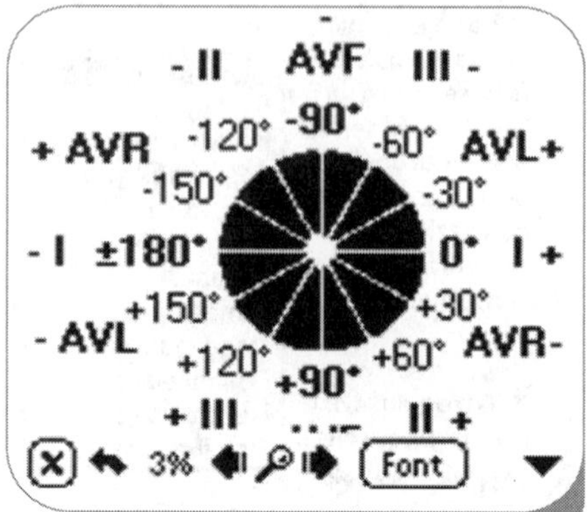

Figure 62B

rescue with this nicely done collection. This document not only lists but also describes each item rather nicely (Figure 63).

The Eponym document also has each letter of the alphabet bookmarked so that you can jump more quickly to that spot. This was a clever idea. Later, you'll see this same applet in the Jfile format, but this one is quite useable too. Actually, Eponyms is available in quite a few different formats, all of them available from the author's web site. Recently, he informed me that the site has posted a "stand-alone" Eponyms product that doesn't require the use of any other reader or database format.

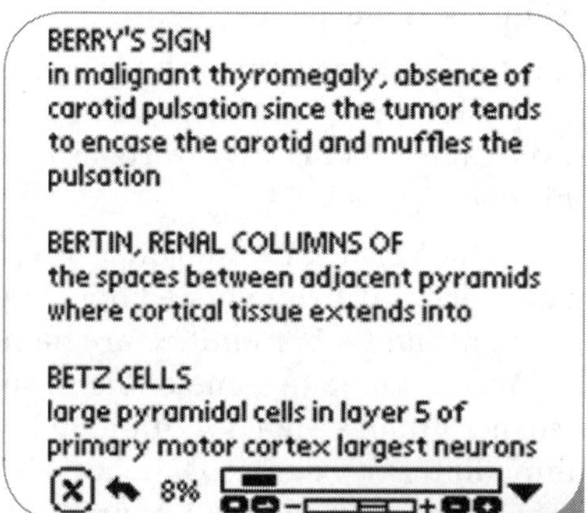

Figure 63

This is definitely worth checking out (see http://eponyms.net for updates or contact Dr. Yee at yee@post.harvard.edu.

7. First Aid Information (46K), by Mary Jo Sminkey (www.dogpatch.org or www.dogpatch.org/email.cfm) and Irish Emergency Ambulance Services Resource, 1998. I like this little document for its simplicity. It does not try to do too much, but covers a limited amount succinctly and well. Admittedly, this piece lacks the depth and sophistication that are required by most medical professionals. However, sometimes a fast, simple, lay answer is needed. This serves that purpose and seems to be a credible source. Here is a sample page from the bookmarks, which provide handy access to all of the included topics and a sample of the text you will see if you tap on Bites, Animal (Figure 64).

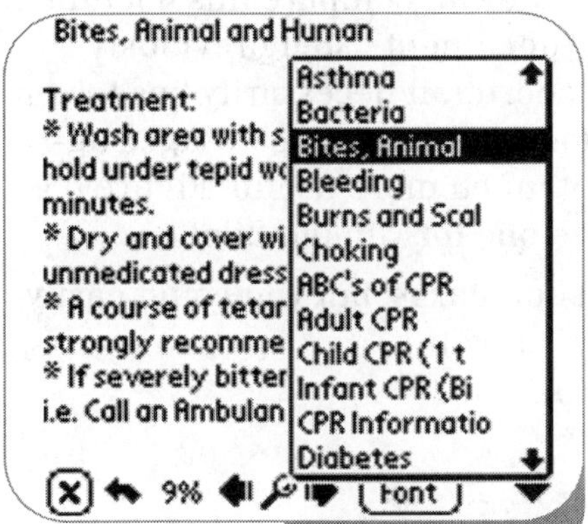

Figure 64A

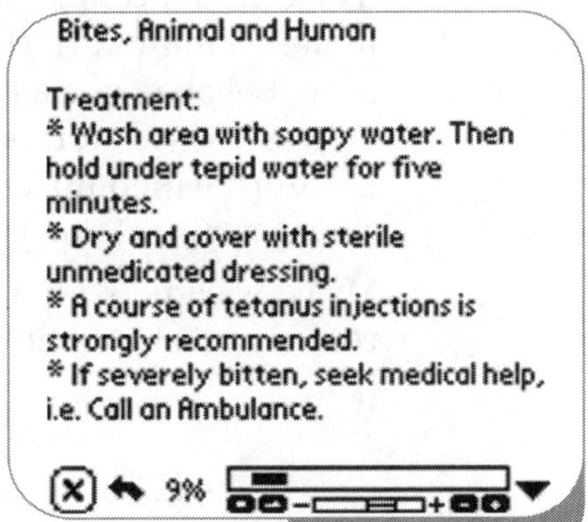

Figure 64B

8. Folstein Mini Mental Status Exam (1K). Ironically, here is a handy memory aid for a brief mental status exam that features memory testing. I find it reassuring that as my memory worsens, I have such resources in my PDA—now if I could just remember where I put my PDA. This obviously brief document has all that it needs from questions and script to scoring. The source and date of this version are unknown, but this is easily checked against the original Folstein.

9. glasgow coma scale [sic] (0K). Similar to the Folstein mentioned previously, this is a short and simple reference. Although it is probably most helpful to the student, any medical professional who frequents the emergency department would find this useful. Once again, author and date of this version are unknown (and I would have capitalized GCS).

10. Herbal Reference Guide (7K). According to the author, "This guide is based on the pharmacy continuing education module called Popular Herbs in the U.S. Market: Therapeutic Monographs (http://www.herbalgram.org/education/conted/popherbs.html), produced and copyrighted by the American Botanical Council." That's a mouthful in order to say that this seems like a credible source, although I'm unsure of the date. Again, I think that this kind of information is increasingly important for discussions with our patients (who are increasingly using herbal remedies). You can compare this document to the "Common Herbs" document listed previously here. Because it is a bit shorter, it necessarily has fewer entries; however, this document contains dosage suggestions, which makes it much more useful. Figure 65 shows a typical entry, the one for Ginkgo Biloba.

    My copy came with no bookmarks, but you could easily remedy this by adding your own.

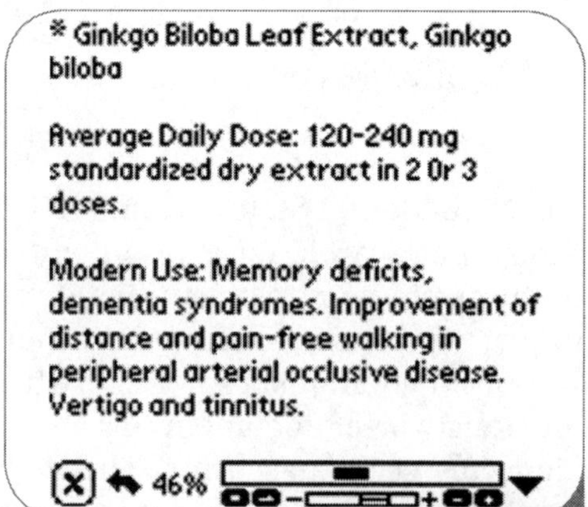

Figure 65

11. ICD-9 Codes for Family Practice (11K), by Kent E. Willyard, M.D. (Compiled by Allen Daugird, M.D., M.B.A., and Donald Spencer, M.D., M.B.A., Department of Family Medicine, University of North Carolina, Chapel Hill. Originally published in Family Practice Management, October 1998. Used with permission.) When considering that the entire ICD-9 code list consists of thousands of entries, you can imagine how limited a document of this size could be. However, the convenience of a short list of "most common" presentations is not to be underestimated. At least this illustrates the importance of having such a reference in a handheld. Commercial PDA solutions for the ICD-9 problem are available, some of them much more extensive (discussed later here). For now, this is concise, free, and useable in your document reader. As I have said, you will see Dr. Willyard's name come up frequently regarding PDA solutions. Here he has thoughtfully added many convenient bookmarks to streamline the process for the user (Figure 66).

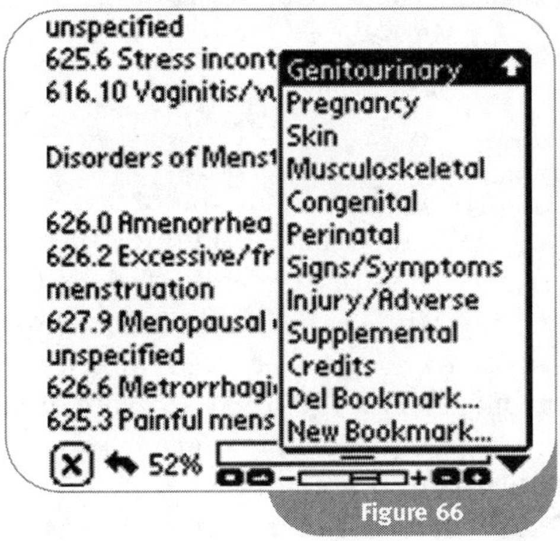

Figure 66

12. List of Phobias (0K). All right, this little document is more for fun, but it could actually be useful too. Did you know the name for the fear of mice? Author and source are unknown.

13. MiniMedMicro (copyright 1999 by e-Med Tools). I list this under Medical Freeware/Shareware because that's the version I have. This software uses a common

scheme among commercial offerings: You get an abridged version free and the full version if you purchase it. Nonetheless, a large amount of useful reference information is available here. I did not list the size of the document because, more properly, MiniMedMicro is a suite of documents (e.g., M2Micro-Fungi [15K], M2Micro-Parasites [12K], M2Micro-Viruses [17K], and M2Micro-Bacteria [unregistered version 11K]). The bookmark section of the latter is shown in Figure 67.

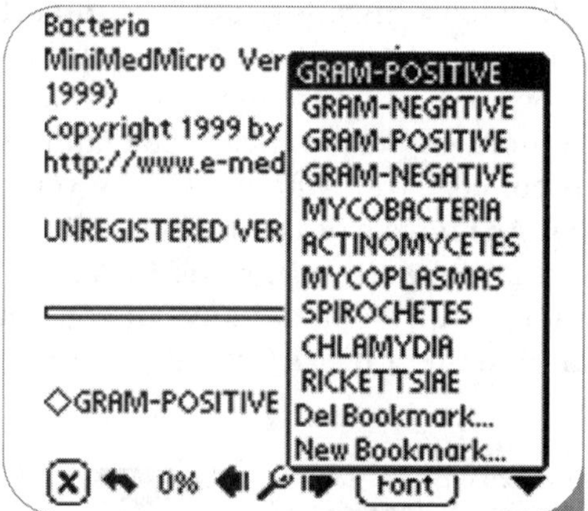

Figure 67

Oddly, only the Fungi document is without bookmarks, leaving it the least user friendly. As I have said, these seem to be good reference materials. Unfortunately, it seems that MiniMedMicro is one of those mysteries of PDA software. Perhaps e-MedTools has divested itself of this property since 1999. At any rate, it is no longer listed at their web site. Several searches showed that it is available from the ZDnet web site (still the 1999 version for $15), but trying to download it was fruitless. I finally did a Google search and was directed to the TuCows site, where I was recently able to download the original document.

14. Musculoskeletal Exam (1K). This is a brief outline for the clinician that even includes bookmarks. Unfortunately, it's another PDA software mystery with unknown source and author.

15. NANDA by Disorders 2.0 (23K), by Tim Warner. These are nursing diagnoses by disorder and seem to include some useful signs and symptoms. Tips are at the bottom of the document, which suggest lookups using the search (find) function, as this document seems to be in no specific order and has no bookmarks.

16. Neurological Exam (0K). This is the briefest of outlines that should serve as a useful reminder for clinicians and students. Even for such a brief document, it manages to include handy bookmarks for cranial nerves, motor, and sensory. Author and source are unknown.

17. On Call: Floor Emergencies (14K), by Kent E. Willyard, M.D. Symptoms, differential diagnoses, etiology, treatments . . . they're all here for the most common serious problems that are likely to confront clinicians on call. Once again, Kent Willyard has presented a very useful tool and has made it user friendly with handy bookmarks.

18. Peripheral Neuro Exam (0K). This is another handy, brief outline for medical professionals. It covers everything from the neck down in a very short but useful manner. The author and source are unknown.

19. pfts (3K). This is a succinct little guide to pulmonary function tests, the breathless patient, spirometry, and more. Although it seems quite useful, it would have been handier with bookmarks. You could add them yourself, however. The author and source are unknown.

20. Sample Floor Notes (4K), by Kent E. Willyard, M.D. By now you should have realized that one of the more prolific clinicians to post useful software on the web is this author, one of my heroes. I love this document. I wish I had this at my fingertips when I was in physician assistant school. Whether you need a reminder about the typical format for an Admit note, an Op note, a Procedure note, or a Discharge note, they're all here and more, with handy bookmarks to take you right to them. I'll admit that when I was new at dictation, I kept a little "cheat sheet" handy. This just seems so much better (and more professional).

21. The Full Physical (4K), by Dr. Pilot Software. If you guessed that it was unlikely that the full physical exam could be reviewed in any meaningful way in just 4K of memory, you would probably be right. This is actually the demo of a commercial product offering and only includes the Cardiovascular and Neurological exams; however, that's okay for a freebie, and it gives you a good feel for the rest of the topics (which are listed in the bookmarks). The Dr. Pilot Software people must be from Canada because their S3 is "Montreal" and their S4 is "Toronto." I thought they were "Tennessee" and "Kentucky."

22. Vitamins and Minerals (9K). The author and source are unknown, but this is a quite thorough job and about what you would expect for a document of this size. It covers everything from calcium to zinc and all of the vitamins, too, with handy bookmarks to take you to each one.

Other useful medical freeware/shareware documents are undoubtedly appearing weekly, but this should give you a good start and a good idea of why PDAs have become so useful in medicine. However, other formats with good medical applets exist as well, and now we look at some of these.

iSilo Files

iSilo is another amazing document reader for the Palm OS handheld. It can read most of the other document files listed previously here but has the advantage of being able to read other iSilo files, which are readable in only iSilo. You may want to try out more than one reader to see which one suits you best. You may also find that you like the available applets for one better than the other. On the other hand, like me, you may find that no one reader will get the entire job done for you: You might like applets that are available in different formats and thus want to have them all. Some documents just read better with different programs. It should also be noted that a freeware version of iSilo is also available. Because it is free, it does not have all of the features of the registered commercial version. As a result, some of the documents listed here do not work as well with the iSilo free version. Here are a few more useful and interesting iSilo medical documents.

- Asthma Meister (44K), by A. Schechtman, 2001 (www.FPPalm.com).

This very good reference and good-sized document is quite navigable with iSilo. It has bookmarks and links built in so that tapping on a particular link within the text takes you to the related information. It includes diagnosis, management of exacerbations, management of chronic asthma, medications, and treatment during pregnancy. All of this is free! It's worth checking out the web site, too, for more in the "Meister" series, such as CodeMeister, LyteMeister, CPT Meister, and more.

- Clinical Dermatology: Demo (48K), by Carl G. Weber, M.D., Internal Medicine, edited by Gary S. Novatt, M.D., Dermatologist (available from http://cgwebermd.tripod.com/Clinical-med).

This is actually a commercial applet, with the full version being $10. Nevertheless, the demo version is pretty good, too, if it happens to have the item for which you are looking. As you can see from Figure 68, this page of the table of contents shows subjects included in the demo version in bold type. Regular type indicates subjects covered in only the full version. This is one of approximately 30 separate titles available. You should definitely check out the web site.

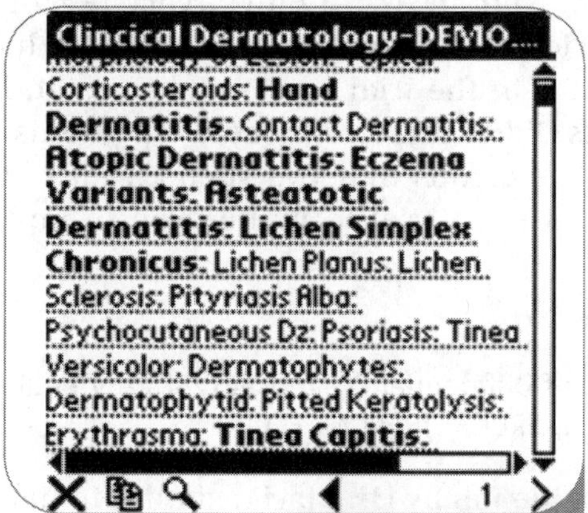

Figure 68

■ Current Medical Therapeutics (47K), by Paul E. Marik, M.D., FCP (SA), M.Med, FRCP (C), FCCM, FCCP 2000 (pmarik@zbzoom.net).

This is a great free text covering the treatments for pulmonary, cardiac, GI, CNS, ID, and metabolic diseases and conditions in an outline synopsis format. Each of the main topic areas just listed are in the table of contents and are bookmarked for ease of use. For easier and quicker navigability, links are built in to the text.

■ DVT Px (2K): DVT Prophylaxis, by Paul Marik, M.D.

This is a very brief but useful document by the same author as the previous item. It includes notes on five Risk Groups with bookmarks to each of them.

■ EBM ICU Protocols (Evidence Based Critical Care Medicine: Balancing the Evidence) (3K), by Paul Marik, M.D.

This is more of a brief article or editorial, but deserves review.

■ Infectious diseases trial (60K), by PDA Medical Solutions, 2000.

This is a very truncated trial version of a commercial product. As usual, it gives a very thorough index, which includes organisms and treatment, infectious diseases and treatment, and antimicrobial treatment, but allows you access to only a very few of the index items in the trial version. You would have to be quite lucky to find what you're looking for in the trial version as a result. It is also too bad that the authors didn't indicate by bold type items that were in the trial version. This means that you spend a lot of time with no results. I guess it's a fair trial to induce you to buy the commercial offering.

■ Marik's Primer of Differential Diagnosis (28K), by Paul Marik, M.D., F.C.P.(S.A.), M.Med, FRCP (C), FCCM, FCCP

This is another fine job by Dr. Marik, similar to his Current Medical Therapeutics (discussed previously here). This text has Cardiology,

Pulmonary, GI, Renal, CNS, Metabolic and Electrolyte, Endocrinology, Hematology, and Miscellaneous, all bookmarked and linked within the text.

■ Ortho trial (76K). PDA Medical Solutions, 2000

This is the truncated trial version of the full commercial version. The trial version includes only one active section (Paediatrics) of a possible five. The inactive sections are General, Regional, Disease, and Trauma. The trial version could still be useful in a pediatric setting, and could quite possibly induce you to purchase the full version.

■ Surgical Knots, Sutures, and Stitches trial (112K). PDA Medical Solutions, 2000

This is another truncated trial version. This one shows you the entire table of contents, but only one of the eleven chapters is active—Chapter 5, Common Suturing Techniques. Although the chapter is active, it does not let you see its illustrations, which makes for a fair demo, but a less useful freebie.

HanDbase Files

HanDbase (available at www.ddhsoftware.com) was mentioned previously in the databases section. Database programs for the PDA do great and useful things with lists of items. Here we review some of the freeware/shareware available for the HanDbase format. This seems to be one of the more fruitful database programs for those in medicine. This could be because developers enjoy working in the format. The newest version, HanDbase 3.0, has just been released and has even more user-friendly features and formatting. Most of the applets reviewed here are available for free at the company's web site, in the gallery section.

■ ACLS Lists (9K), Author unknown.

This seems to be a useful applet of only nine items. It's not the best use of HanDbase or the user-friendliest applet, but it does show you the potential of the database. Figure 69 shows a screen shot of the nine items.

If you tap on "PVC's," for example, you will come to the record screen for PVCs (Figure 70).

This is how records are edited and viewed. If you tap on the "Notes," you will come to the core of this applet, as shown in Figure 71.

More information is available in the note, as indicated by the control arrow at the right side of the page. This is not particularly exciting but is illustrative and appears useful. I would feel better if I knew the author and source material.

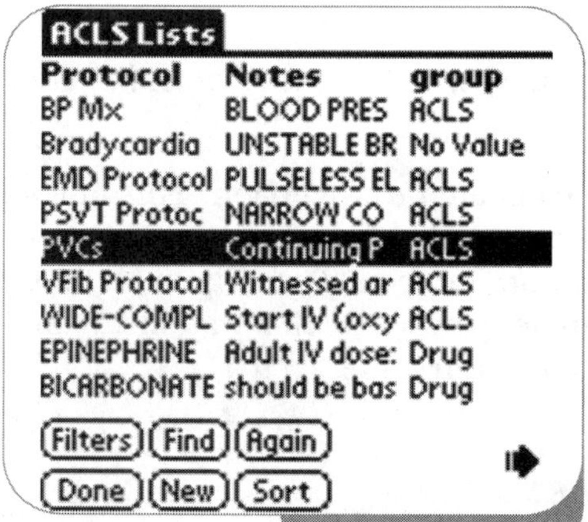

Figure 69

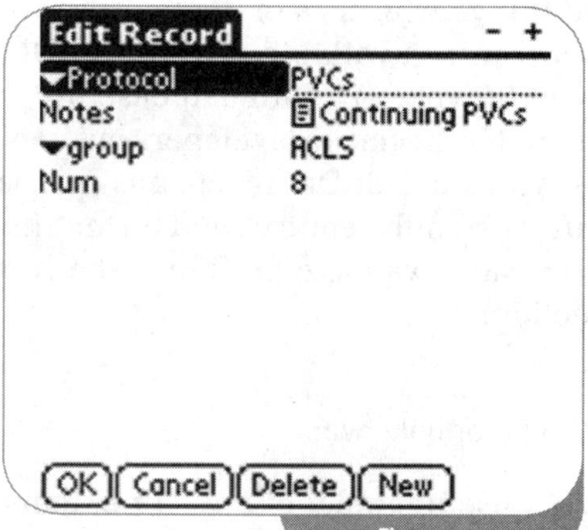
Edit Record
Protocol PVCs
Notes Continuing PVCs
group ACLS
Num 8
OK Cancel Delete New

Figure 70

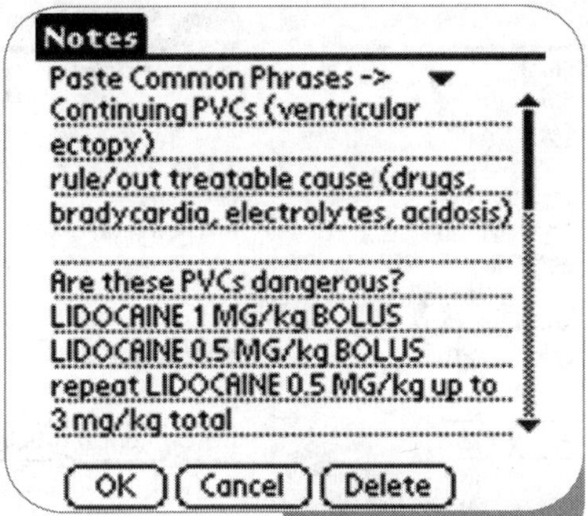

Figure 71

■ Alticopeia (125K), by David Rappaport.

This is a much finer example of the power of a database and the ease of use of HanDbase. David Rappaport has done a stellar job here. The size of the applet is reflective of the number of entries in it. Take a look at just one page, as shown in Figure 72.

This is just the beginning of the As! If we tap on Aloe, we come to the data record of Aloe that takes up two pages (Figure 73).

Many individual records are contained in this applet, which makes this a very useful tool. You'll also notice the controls at the bottom of the first screen shot (Figure 72) "Find" and "Sort." These are functions that

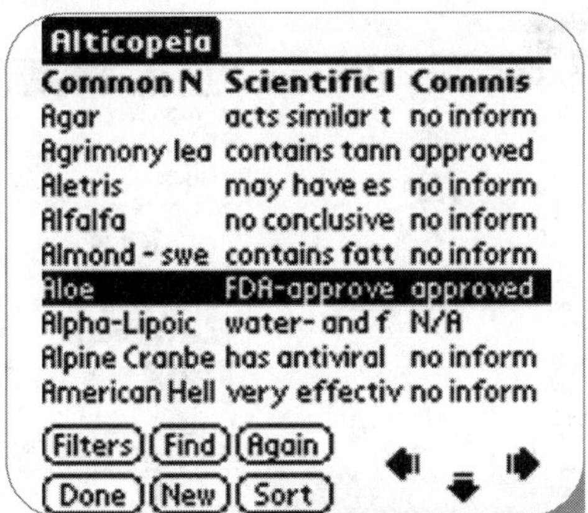
Alticopeia
Common N Scientific I Commis
Agar acts similar t no inform
Agrimony lea contains tann approved
Aletris may have es no inform
Alfalfa no conclusive no inform
Almond - swe contains fatt no inform
Aloe FDA-approve approved
Alpha-Lipoic water- and f N/A
Alpine Cranbe has antiviral no inform
American Hell very effectiv no inform
Filters
Find
Again
Done
New
Sort
Figure 72

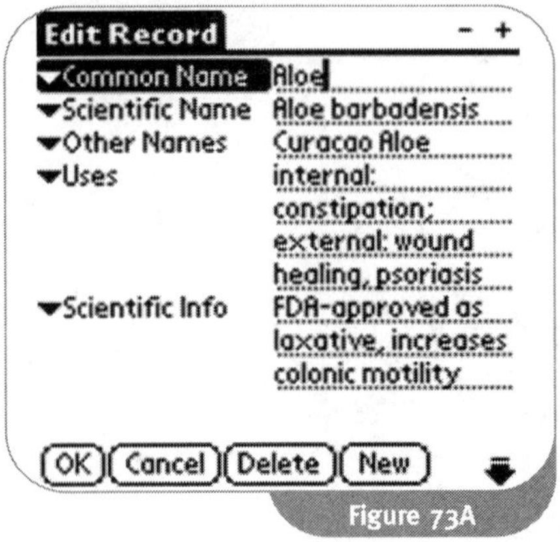
Edit Record
- +
Common Name Aloe
Scientific Name Aloe barbadensis
Other Names Curacao Aloe
Uses internal: constipation; external: wound healing, psoriasis
Scientific Info FDA-approved as laxative, increases colonic motility
OK Cancel Delete New
Figure 73A

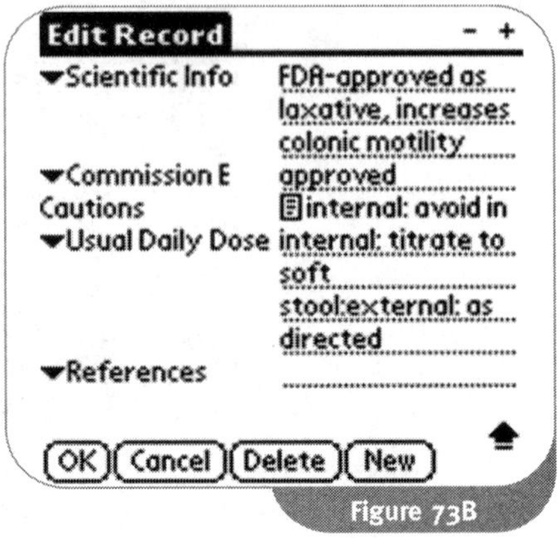
Edit Record
- +
Scientific Info FDA-approved as laxative, increases colonic motility
Commission E approved
Cautions internal: avoid in
Usual Daily Dose internal: titrate to soft stool;external: as directed
References
OK Cancel Delete New
Figure 73B

make the database even quicker to use. With tools like this, you don't have to scroll through the entire list to find what you need. These tools deserve some experimentation on your part to get familiar with them. Mastering them will save a lot of time.

■ Antibiotic Efficacies (7K), author unknown.

Because the author, date and source of this applet are unknown, I wouldn't recommend this as a reference. I include it here because it once more illustrates potential. In addition, it seems like this would be a useful template for anyone who wanted to take the time to insert his or her own local resistance patterns on a timely basis (Figure 74).

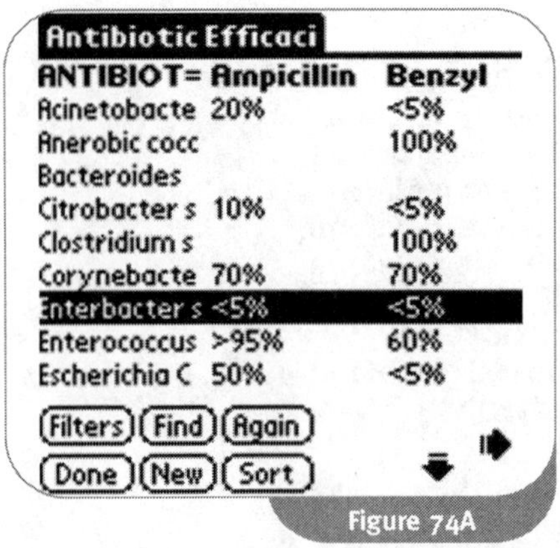

Figure 74A

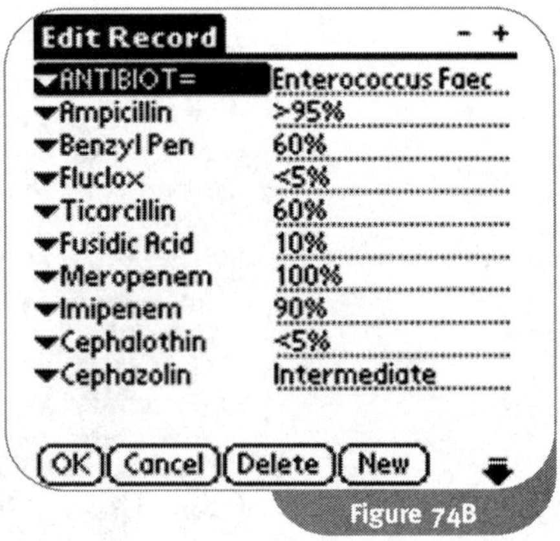

Figure 74B

Here we see a page sorted by infectious organism. If we tap on "Enterococcus," we come to the record screen for Enterococcus that indicates the efficacy for various antibiotics. Notes and source would also have been helpful.

■ APGAR Score (3K), by Richard Dabbs (rdabbs@usa.net).

This is a neat, small applet that does only one thing, but does it well. This shows an interesting side to HanDbase. The author has actually used the calculate function to build this applet. In other words, when the user enters information into this applet, it automatically calculates the APGAR score for the patient. What's more, you can calculate and save the data on many patients. This would be handy, for example, on pediatric rounds. In Figure 75, you see the opening screen for a new record. Here you would enter the patient's name, use the drop down menus to quickly insert the date and time, and then choose between a 1- and 5-minute APGAR.

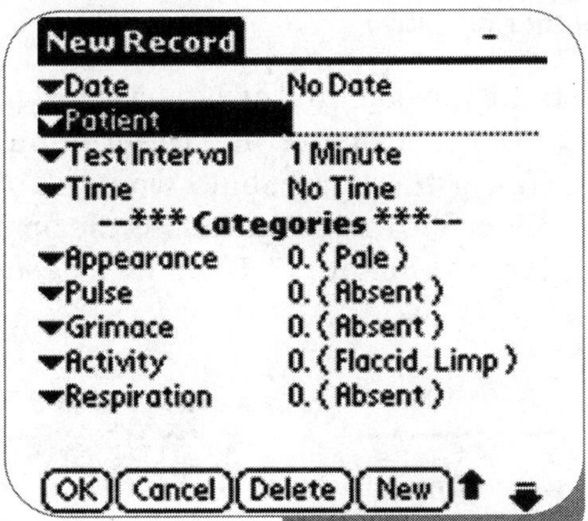

Figure 75

In the Categories section are the five APGAR test categories with a dropdown menu for each one. If you tap on the arrow next to Appearance, for example, you get the menu shown in Figure 76

The user then would tap on the appropriate choice from the menu. After choosing one choice from each menu (one per category), the

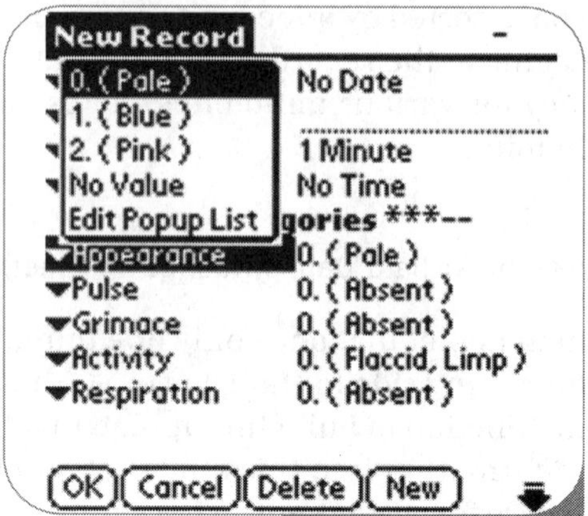

Figure 76

program calculates the APGAR score and records it. Nicely done. The author tells me an improved version is coming soon.

- Bones (31K), author unknown.

This applet also shows the potential of database programs. It only consists of three fields: Bone, Structure, and Description, which is all that is needed. I don't know the source, but I wouldn't be surprised if all of the bones were here. Shown in Figure 77 is the opening screen shot (77A), the record for the capitate (77B), and its description (77C).

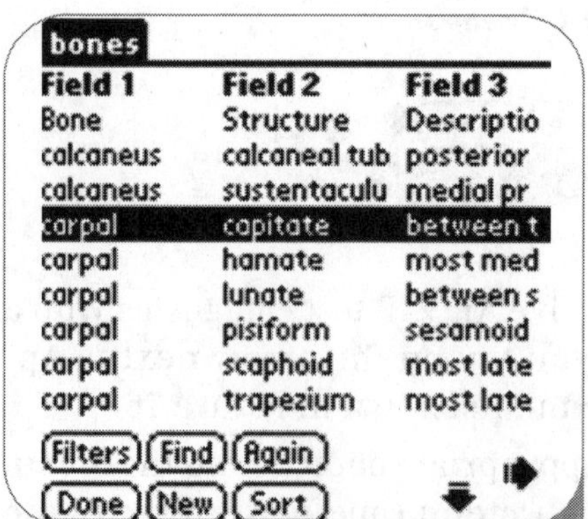

Figure 77A

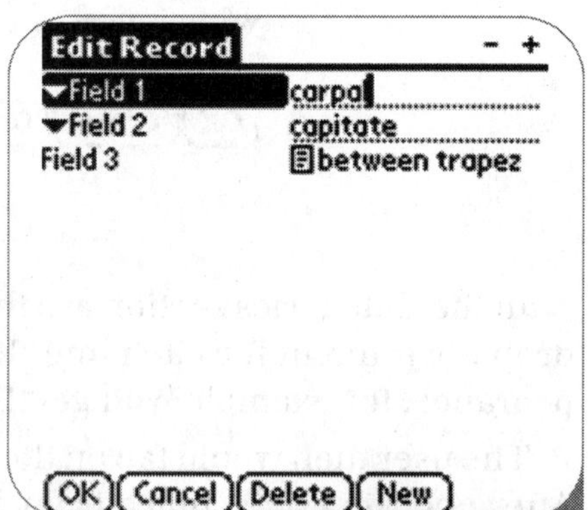

Figure 77B

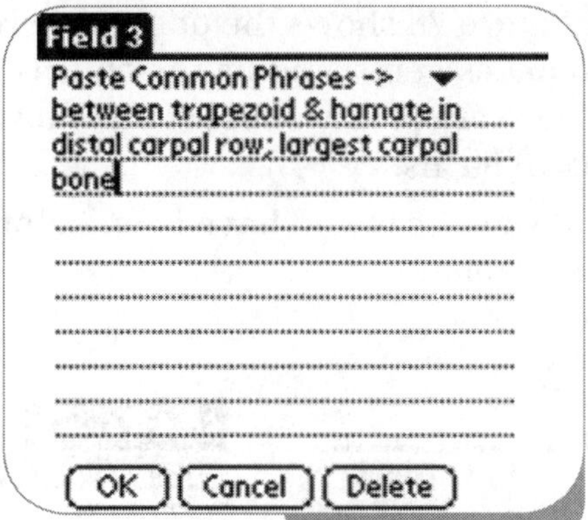

Figure 77C

■ Chest Discomfort (24K), by Brad Klein (med2be@hotmail.com).

This interesting applet organizes your thinking about the differential diagnosis of chest discomfort. The database can be sorted by cause, general category, or other parameters to make it more user friendly. This one deserves your attention.

■ CPT Codes (4K), by Charles Southerland, DPM, FACFAS.

This applet is, again, just illustrative. A colleague, podiatrist Dr. Charles Southerland, has devised this short database of CPT codes applicable to podiatric medicine. Consisting of only two fields, it includes the code and the description. You can easily imagine the usefulness of being able to sort the list by either code or description and having those codes handy. In fact, Dr. Southerland has incorporated this database into a patient-tracking database for podiatric surgical residents. Many possibilities exist with databases.

■ Electrolyte ddx (8K), author unknown.

This interesting applet has more fields than it takes advantage of most of the time. Its intent is to derive a differential diagnosis for various electrolyte disturbances. It seems to me, however, that it works better backward. Figure 78 shows the opening screen shot and then the following two pages generated by the "burns" database record. You can see that there are plenty of fields that may be better used for other diagnoses than burns.

Instructions and sources would have been helpful, but this is nevertheless a useful template.

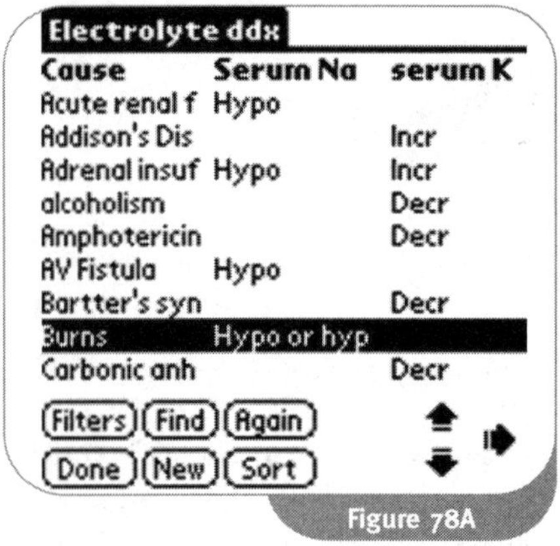

Figure 78A

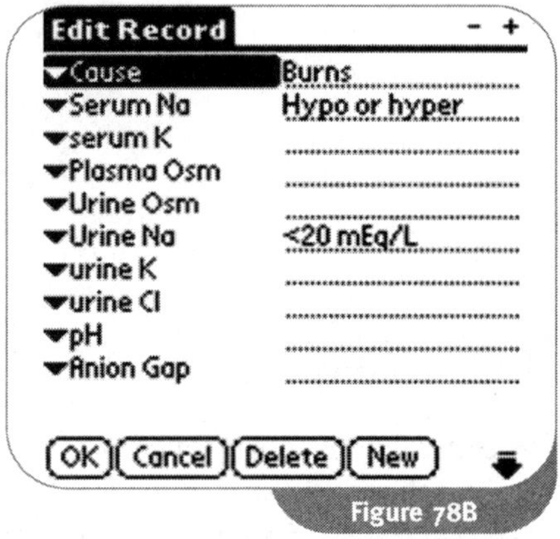

Figure 78B

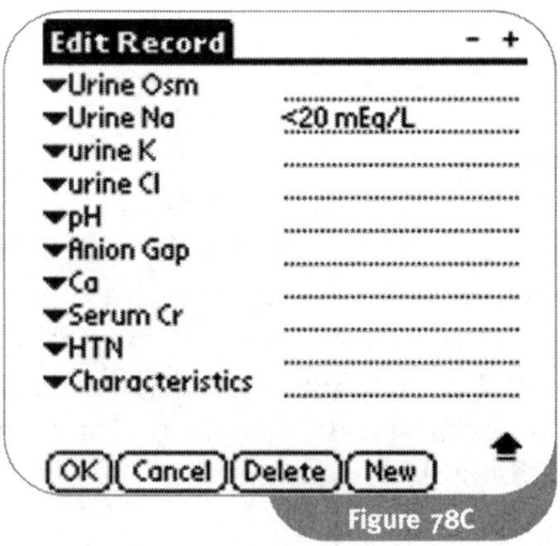

Figure 78C

- Fever and Rash (19K), by Brad Klein (med2be@hotmail.com).

In this interesting applet, the author has put a lot of useful information into an easily accessible database. Figure 79 shows the opening

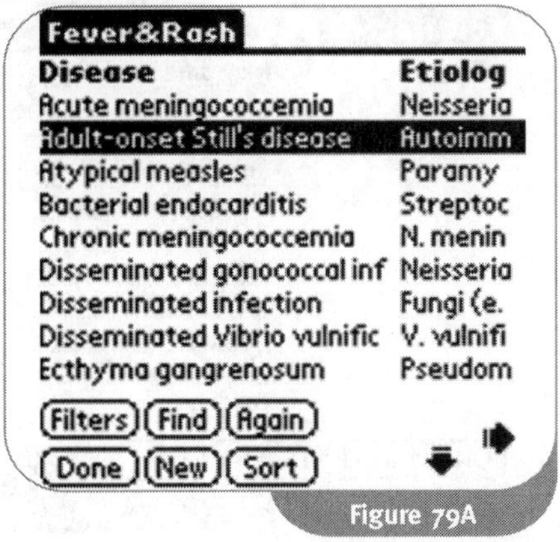

Figure 79A

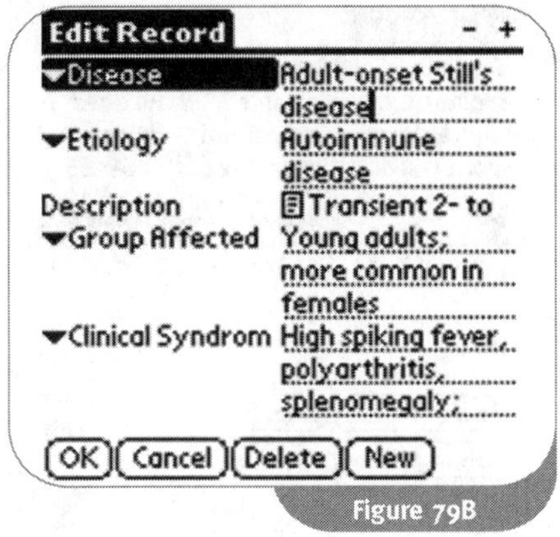
Edit Record
Disease Adult-onset Still's disease
Etiology Autoimmune disease
Description Transient 2- to
Group Affected Young adults; more common in females
Clinical Syndrom High spiking fever, polyarthritis, splenomegaly;
OK Cancel Delete New
Figure 79B

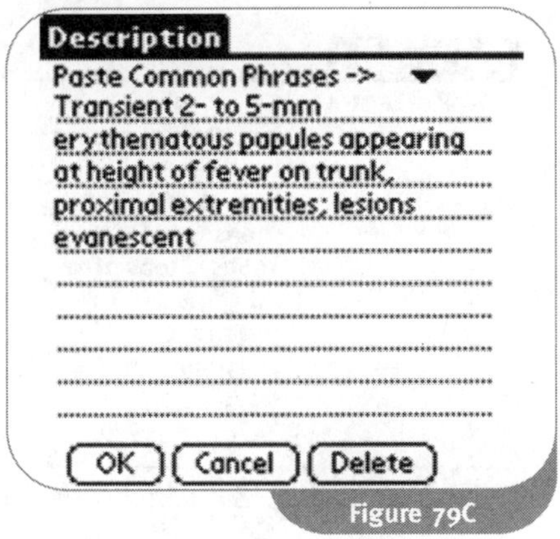

Figure 79C

screen, followed by the record for Adult-onset Still's Disease, and a screen shot showing the expanded description field.

As with most of the HanDbase applets, you could also sort this database by different fields such as etiology or description. This seems to be a quite useful database.

■ Headache (5K), by Brad Klein (med2be@hotmail.com).

Here is another useful applet from a frequent HanDbase contributor. It lists only six possible headache types but gives good information. Figure 80 shows the opening screen shot with the records sorted by headache type and screen shots of the two pages of the migraine record.

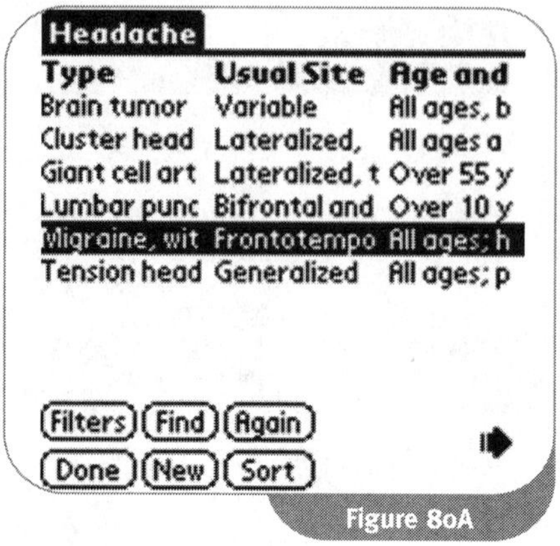

Figure 8oA

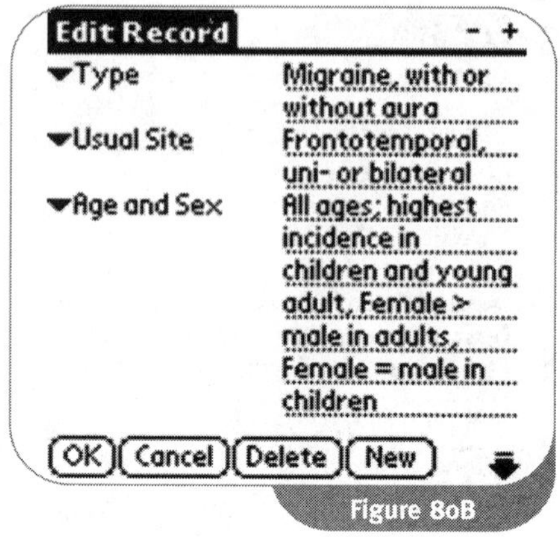
Edit Record
Type Migraine, with or without aura
Usual Site Frontotemporal, uni- or bilateral
Age and Sex All ages; highest incidence in children and young adult. Female > male in adults. Female = male in children
OK Cancel Delete New

Figure 8oB

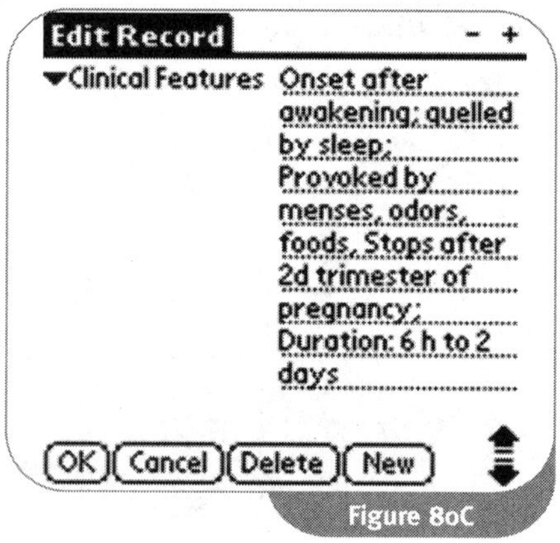
Edit Record
Clinical Features Onset after awakening; quelled by sleep; Provoked by menses, odors, foods. Stops after 2d trimester of pregnancy; Duration: 6 h to 2 days
OK Cancel Delete New

Figure 8oC

I would like to see this expanded into even more types and etiologies, but this is useful and would be a good template to which to add your own data.

■ Lab Interpretation (58K), author unknown.

This is a great database even though I don't know the source of the information. It seems we're always faced with interpreting abnormal laboratory results; a guide like this would be a handy place to start. Figure 81 shows the opening screen shot if the database is sorted by laboratory test, followed by a screen shot of the record of the albumin test.

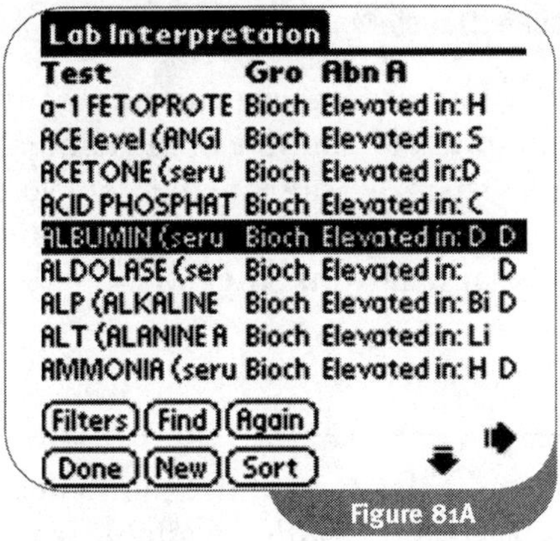

Figure 81A

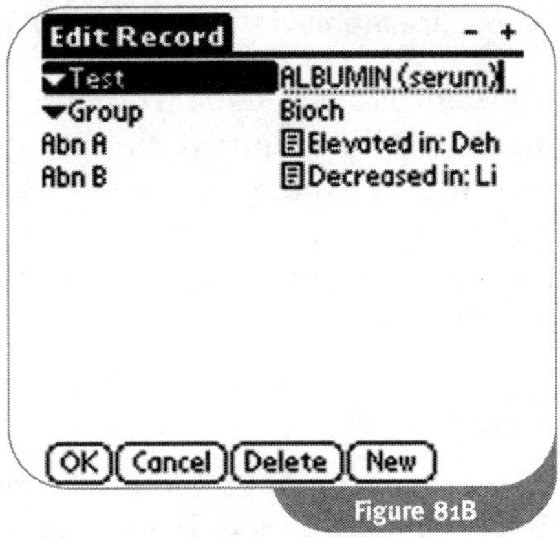

Figure 81B

Because there is usually more information than will fit on a line, the author has added extra fields for abnormal highs and lows. Those two screen shots are shown in Figures 82A and 82B.

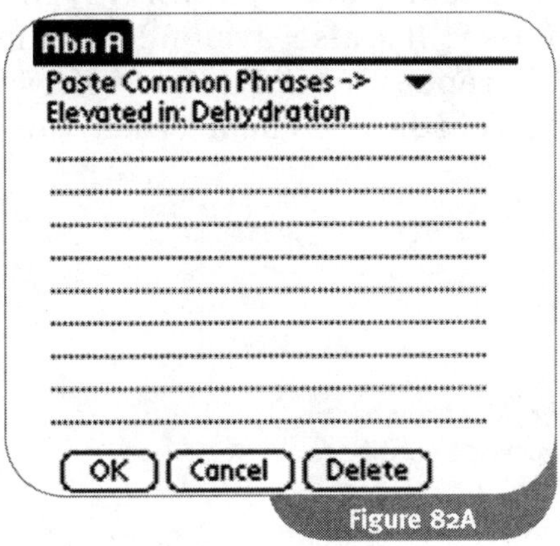

Figure 82A

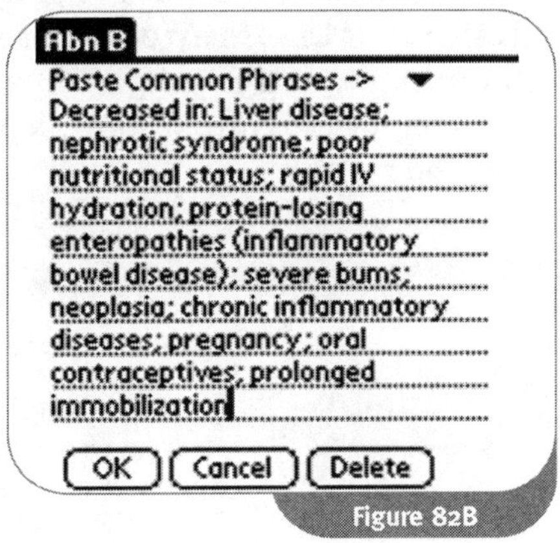

Figure 82B

The database would have been even more useful if normal laboratory values would have been included. Then I could have done all of my looking in one place.

■ LFT (24K), by Brad Klein (med2be@hotmail.com).

Like the author's other databases, this is a simple, useful tool. Records for 16 disease states can be sorted by disease or any of the liver tests (bili, alk phos, aminotransferase, or ALT/AST).

- Medical Abbreviations (22K), by Michael.Dansie@hsc.utah.

This one is a winner. A truly simple and handy database, this has many of the medical abbreviations that you might encounter in the clinical world. The rapid way to use this database is by entering the item you are looking for in the Find function. It can't possibly have everything in just 22K of memory, but it has most of what you'll need.

Jfiles

There's not a whole lot to say about the Jfiles format in the medical realm. Jfiles are documents made to be read with Jfile (available from www.land-j.com) and, to be sure, they have qualities to recommend them. The problem is that currently too few medical documents are available. Maybe developers don't like to write in this format as well as they like to write in others. Nevertheless, some documents are just better viewed in certain formats. Here I would like to make the case for Jfile. You might recall a document called Eponyms (by Andrew Yee, M.D.), reviewed previously. It's also available in the Jfile format, and I compare the differences here. First, to refresh your memory, Figure 83 shows a page from the document format using TealDoc reader.

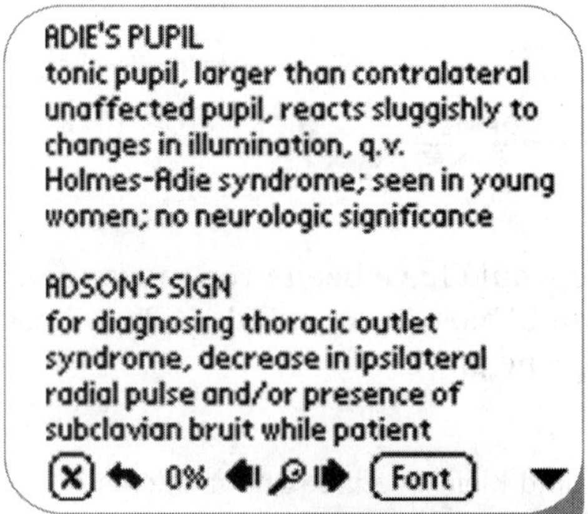

ADIE'S PUPIL
tonic pupil, larger than contralateral unaffected pupil, reacts sluggishly to changes in illumination, q.v. Holmes-Adie syndrome; seen in young women; no neurologic significance
ADSON'S SIGN
for diagnosing thoracic outlet syndrome, decrease in ipsilateral radial pulse and/or presence of subclavian bruit while patient
0%
Font

Figure 83

Figure 84 shows essentially the same page of Eponyms Jfile.

You can see that it is much more easily searched, similar to a database. You would then tap on Adie's pupil to come to the text screen for that entry (Figure 85).

I like this format better for this document, although it might not be preferable for all documents. In addition, as I said, too few medical documents are currently available in this format. Thus, I don't know that I would pay for Jfile just for the sake of the medical offerings. However, as you search web sites such as www.MemoWare.com,

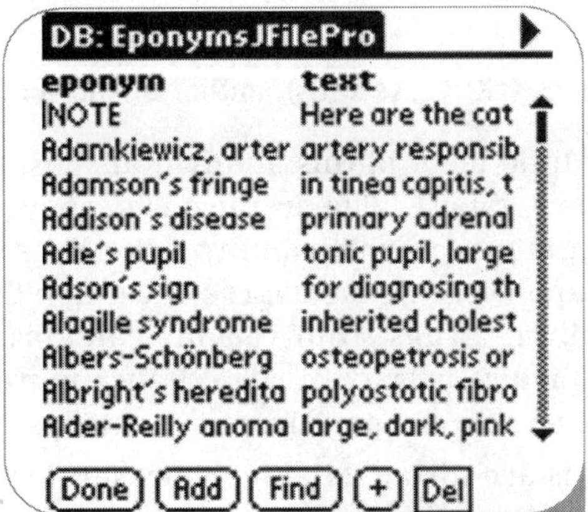

Figure 84

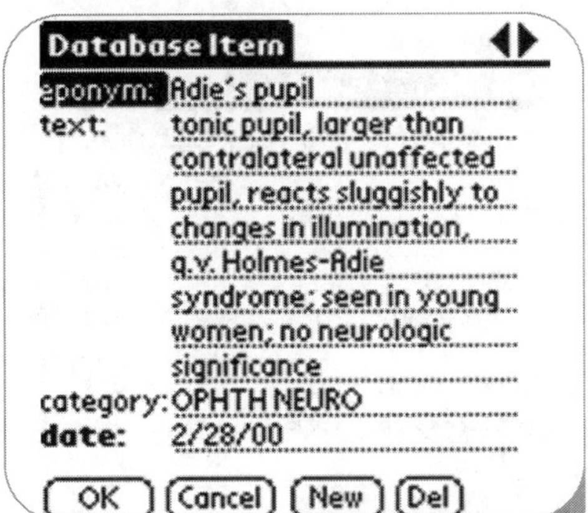

Figure 85

you may see lots of other things popping up that require Jfile and that you just can't live without on your PDA.

MobileDB Files

MobileDB files (which are available at www.mobiledb.com or www.handmark.com) are just a little more abundant for medical topics than the Jfiles. Apparently, developers just like to write in the MobileDB format. Whatever the reason, there are several useful items that should be mentioned here.

- Antihypertensives (2K) (13 records), author unknown.

Although I'm a little leery of this anonymous posting, I like the organization of the database. The premise is to show, in tabular form, 13 different conditions for which antihypertensives might be considered. Then the applet shows the degree of caution that should be applied to prescribing drugs from various categories for the given condition. One picture is truly worth a thousand words in this case, and thus Figure 86 shows a page from the database.

More columns are also available, representing Alpha Blockers and Diuretics. Because the source is not known, I'm not sure that I can recommend the information. The organization is nevertheless convenient.

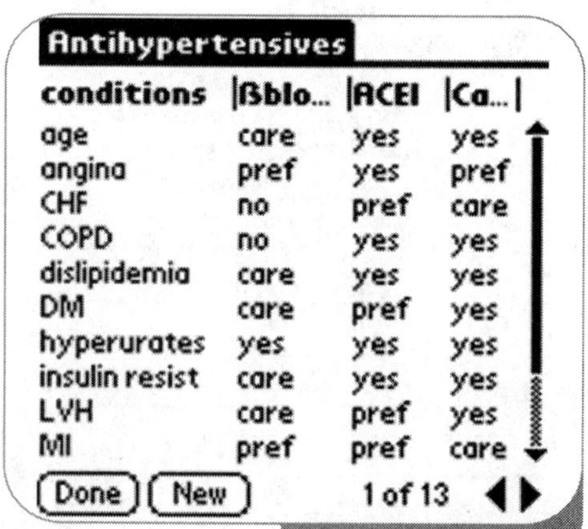
Antihypertensives

conditions	ßblo...	ACEI	Ca...
age	care	yes	yes
angina	pref	yes	pref
CHF	no	pref	care
COPD	no	yes	yes
dislipidemia	care	yes	yes
DM	care	pref	yes
hyperurates	yes	yes	yes
insulin resist	care	yes	yes
LVH	care	pref	yes
MI	pref	pref	care

Done New 1 of 13

Figure 86

■ APA's DSM-IV Codes (30K) (399 records), author unknown.

This simple database packs a fair number of records into a relatively small amount of memory. The basis of this database is reportedly the American Psychiatric Association's Diagnostic and Statistical Manual-IV, although I'm sure that they do not sanction this particular database. This is the type of useful reference for which databases were made.

■ Food Values (92K) (978 records), author unknown.

I love this one. Although not strictly medical, it contains the kinds of information that you need to have at your fingertips to answer patients' questions. I've also used it occasionally to convince my wife that what I was about to eat really would fit into a low-carbohydrate diet. Figure 87 shows a typical page from Food Values and the resulting detail page if we were to tap on Cauliflower.

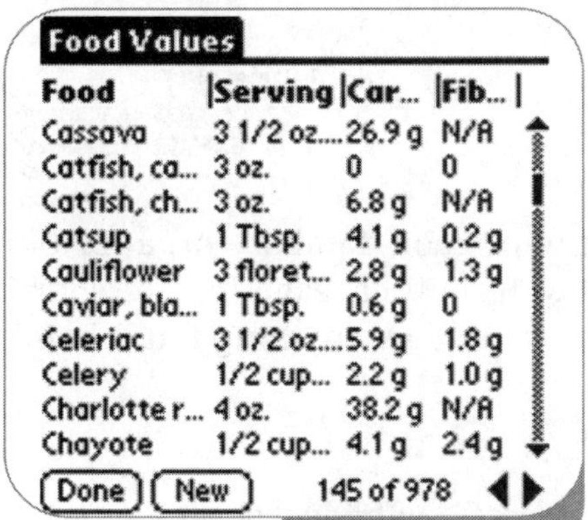
Food Values
Food |Serving |Car... |Fib... |
Cassava 3 1/2 oz.... 26.9 g N/A
Catfish, ca... 3 oz. 0 0
Catfish, ch... 3 oz. 6.8 g N/A
Catsup 1 Tbsp. 4.1 g 0.2 g
Cauliflower 3 floret... 2.8 g 1.3 g
Caviar, bla... 1 Tbsp. 0.6 g 0
Celeriac 3 1/2 oz.... 5.9 g 1.8 g
Celery 1/2 cup... 2.2 g 1.0 g
Charlotte r... 4 oz. 38.2 g N/A
Chayote 1/2 cup... 4.1 g 2.4 g
Done
New
145 of 978

Figure 87A

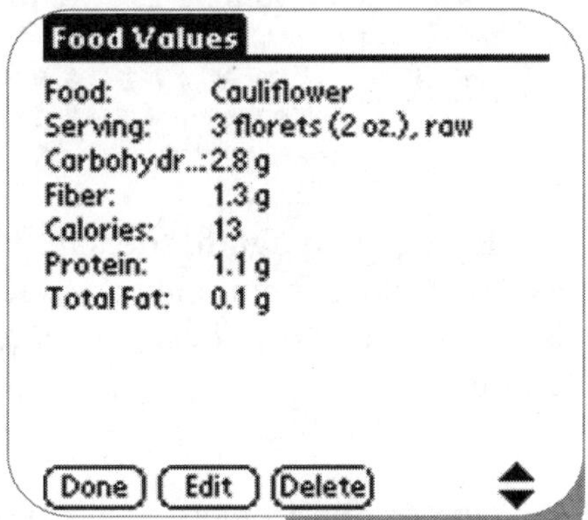
Food Values
Food: Cauliflower
Serving: 3 florets (2 oz.), raw
Carbohydr...: 2.8 g
Fiber: 1.3 g
Calories: 13
Protein: 1.1 g
Total Fat: 0.1 g
Done
Edit
Delete

Figure 87B

You can see that there are several more columns than will fit on the screen. You can use navigation arrows to move over to another column, the lines separating columns to change the column size to a narrower one, or just tap on an item to reveal its entire record. I find that this database, with its large number of records, generally has almost any food item that I am looking for. Even though the source is unknown, the decisions that are made from these data are unlikely to be life threatening anyway. This is very handy.

■ Lab Values 2.0 (10K) (162 records), author unknown.

When you don't use a particular laboratory test frequently, it's good to have a handy reference such as this. With a surprising number of records in a small amount of space, this database packs in a lot of information. You can sort the database by test name or by category, and each test has the normals in both U.S. and SI units. Figure 88 shows a page from the database and the detailed record page that you would see if you tapped on Hgb male.

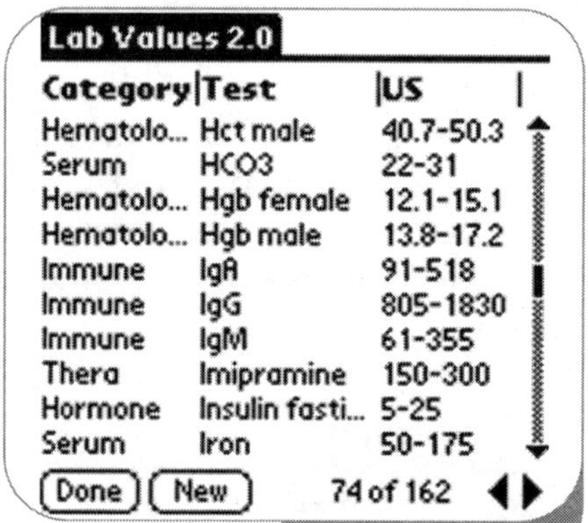

Figure 88A

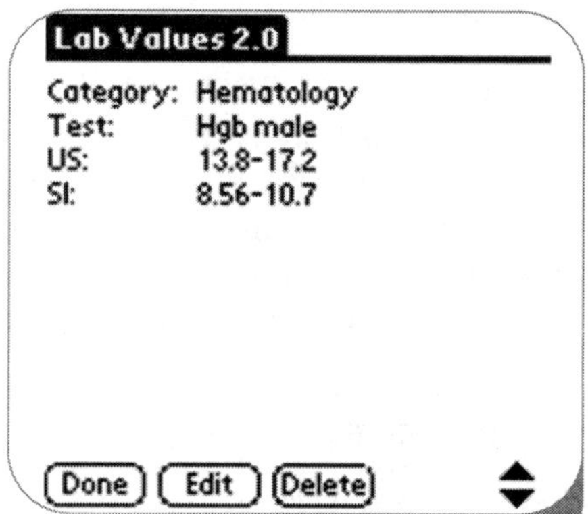

Figure 88B

This is, once again, the same kind of good database organization as Food Values mentioned previously. The only caveat is that the source is unknown. Therefore, I wouldn't use this as anything but a handy guide.

■ Neurological Disorders (153K) (184 records), author unknown.

Although I'm unsure that this is the best use of a database, it is interesting and acts more like a dictionary. Many records and a lot of information, but really only two fields, are here. Figure 89 shows a page from the database and part of the detailed record if we were to tap on Bell's Palsy.

You can see that the findings might go on for several pages, and they usually do. This suggests to me that a different format might have allowed for more information per page. I still like this database for the information that it contains; however, once again, the source is unknown.

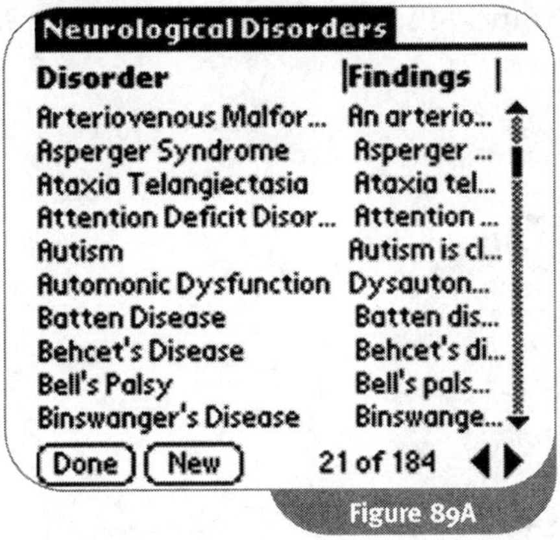

Figure 89A

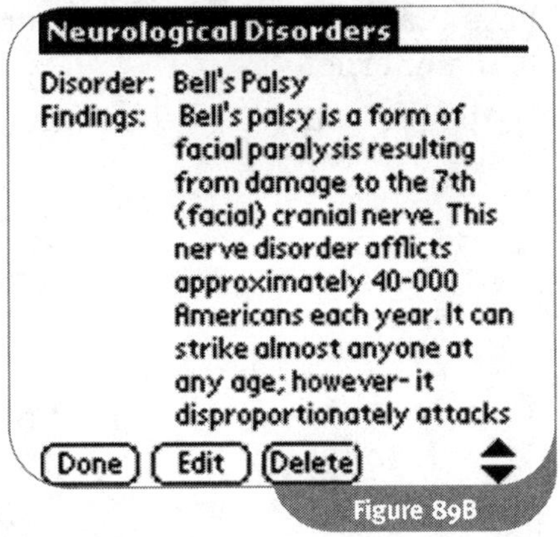

Figure 89B

■ Periodic Table (14K) (109 records), by Ilya Katsnelson.

This isn't strictly a medical database. Nevertheless, we all had to take Chemistry, right? Thus, here is a handy reference that includes all of the elements and quite a few details about each one on the individual record page (Figure 90).

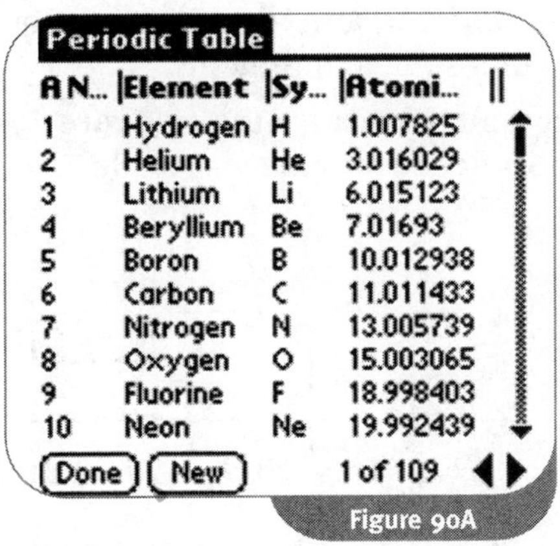

Figure 90A

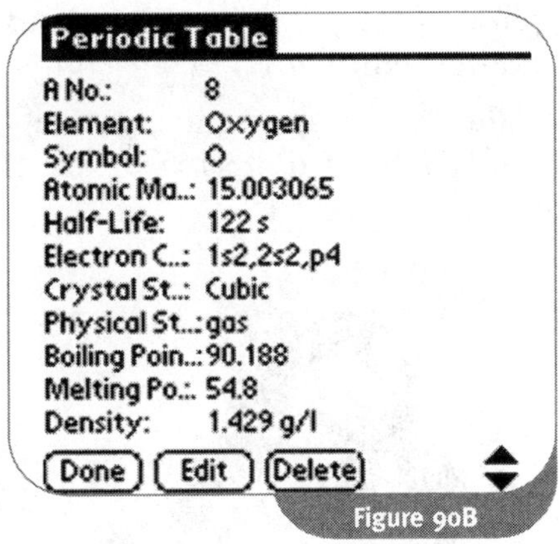

Figure 90B

Images

Ready-made medical images are not too abundant yet. Maybe people are afraid of copyright infringement. A few are worth noting, however. All require one of the image-viewing programs (such as FireViewer). Once you are hooked on carrying around images in your

PDA, maybe you'd like to convert some other images and post them to the Internet.

You previously saw the skull image with labels (Figure 91).

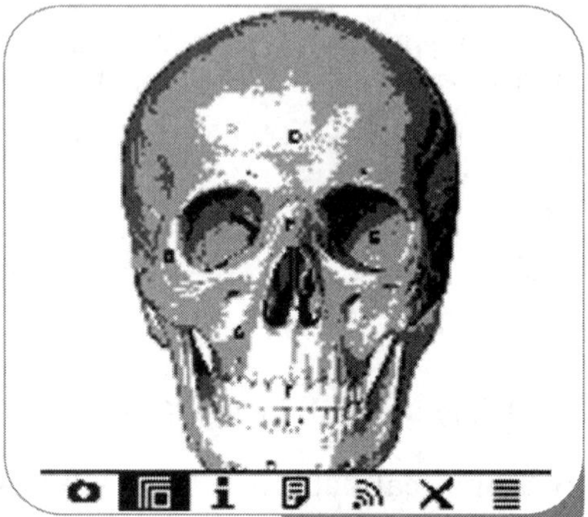

Figure 91

Lateral, top, and posterior views of the skull also exist to go with the frontal. Similarly, there is a series on the knee, an acetaminophen nomogram, an EKG hexaxial diagram, and an acid/base diagram (Figure 92). I'm sure others will also be popping up.

The views shown here are not complete because the software actually allows mobility within the image. You can also reduce or magnify.

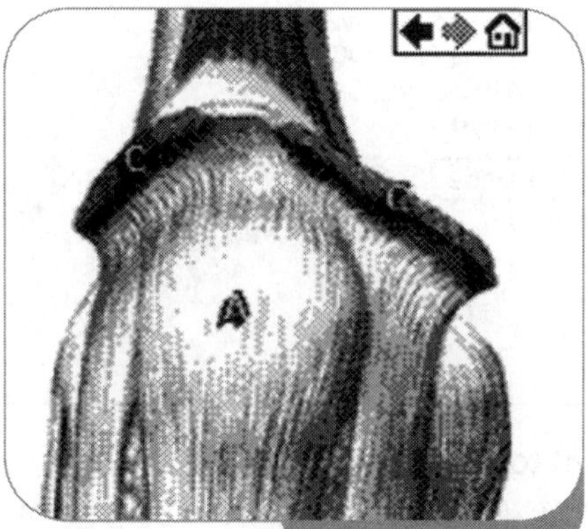

Figure 92A

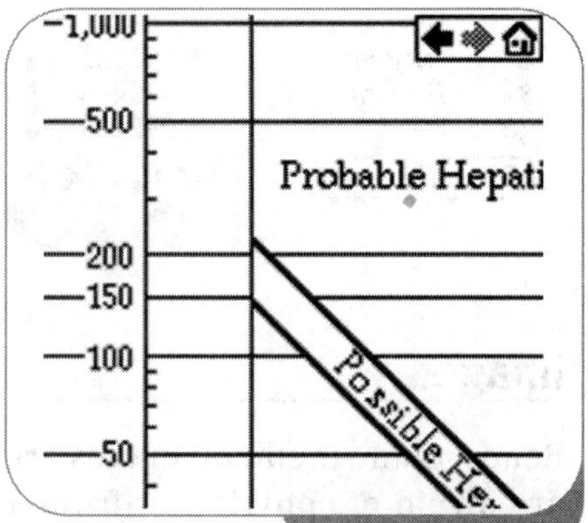

Figure 92B

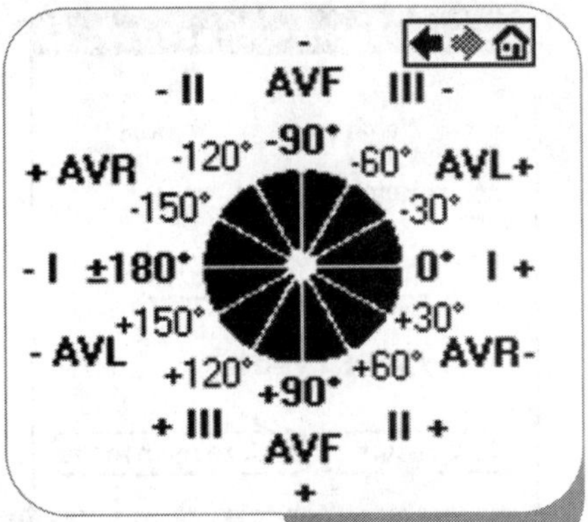

Figure 92C

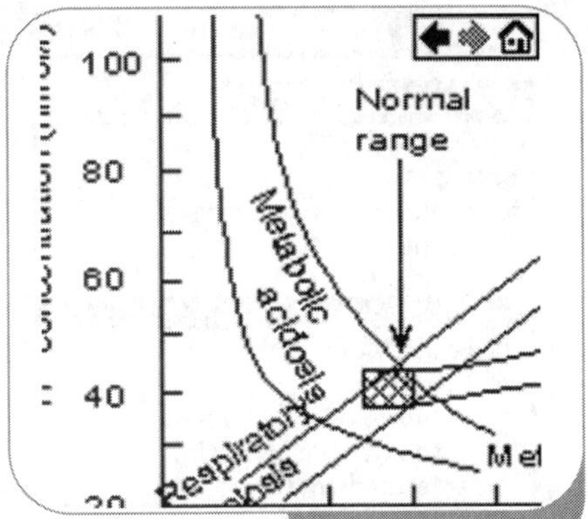

Figure 92D

I wish that it were possible to show you here how your PDA can even turn into a short movie viewer. FireViewer and other programs actually allow you to view short animations. Of course, these little movies consume a lot of memory but are also very impressive. An animated axial dissection from the Visible Human Project is a few seconds long and occupies 1600 K of memory. This may be good for demonstration purposes, but you probably wouldn't want to carry too many of these around in your handheld.

MedCalc/MedMath/Parens/MedRules

The calculator function is certainly one of the most useful functions of the PDA. It gets plenty of use in medicine, but other specialized medical calculators will make your PDA indispensable.

■ MedCalc, by Dr. Mathias Tschopp. My copy (version 2.31) is MedCalc 2000 (99K).

This is an invaluable addition to a medical professional's handheld computer. I counted 36 different equations built into this eminently usable program. Figure 93 shows just one page from the main menu and a detail of what you would see if you tapped on Body surface area.

You have options to select input and output in English or Metric measurements and also have the ability to save the result of any calculation, attribute it to a particular patient, and save it on the Patient

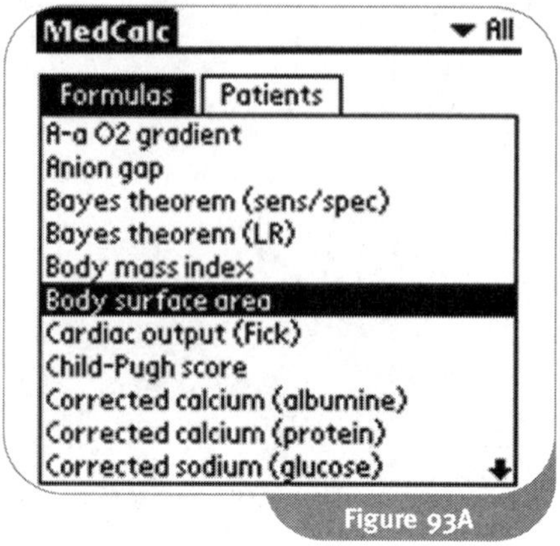

Figure 93A

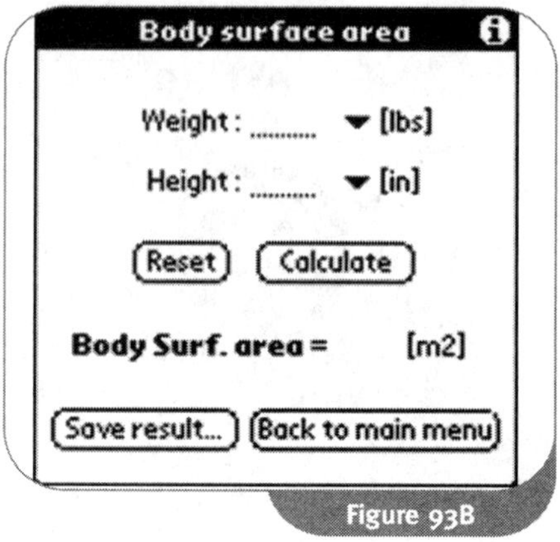

Figure 93B

list page. Calculations are available here that I never dreamed of and others that I have long ago forgotten. Often references are included for the source material. It's nice to have them all in one place. This is a very user-friendly program that I highly recommend.

■ MedMath (37K), Version 1.1 2000, by Phillip Cheng, M.D. (e-mail: pcheng@post.harvard.edu).

This medical calculator is similar to MedCalc. A bit smaller in memory, this has 28 equations. It does away with the patient list feature but includes a handy calculator keyboard on each calculation page. It can also be reset in either English or metric equivalents. Figure 94 shows a page from the main menu of MedMath and a screen shot of one of its calculations.

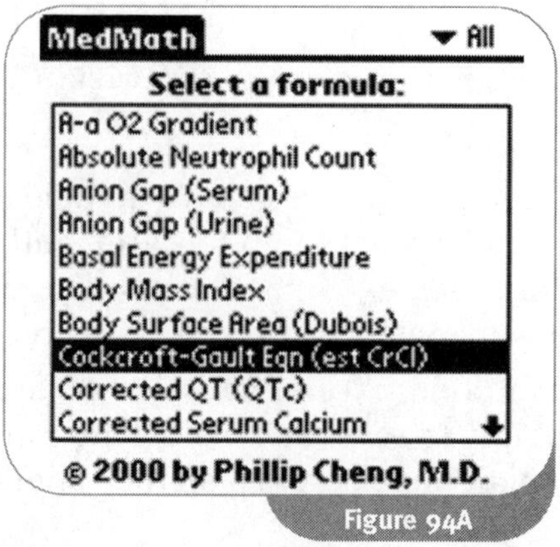

Figure 94A

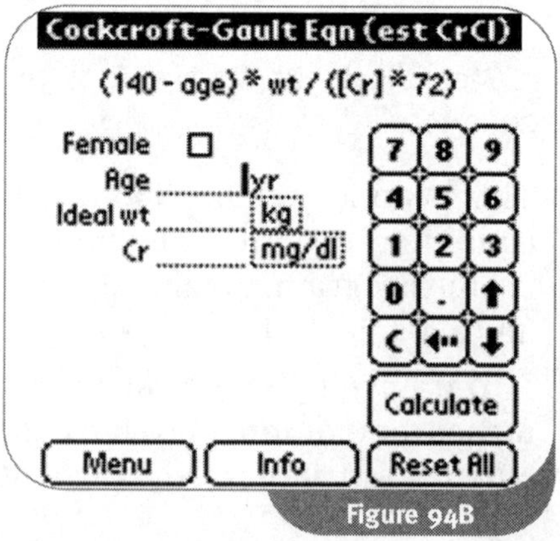

Figure 94B

You should compare the features and equations of these two highly recommended programs to see which one suits your needs more. Interestingly, the folks at ePocrates thought that MedMath was a useful enough tool to include the 2002 version as one of their Med Tools in the ePocrates Pro edition.

- Parens (version 1.3, 1999, by Rick Huebner) (66K) (e-mail: rhuebner

For those of you with a HandSpring-brand PDA, you can ignore this entry. In an earlier section, I talked about the built-in functions of the PDA, and the equivalent of Parens is built in to HandSprings as the advanced calculator. Parens makes your built-in calculator look anemic, as this calculator appears to be on steroids. If you want to make easy English/Metric conversions (among many others), then this is the calculator you want to have installed. It's amazing. Here's what I mean. In Figure 95A, you'll see the opening screen shot of Parens when the option is set to Weight. Figure 95B shows a shot of the dropdown menu choices for other choices than Weight. You can see that the calculator could easily be switched over to Length, for example.

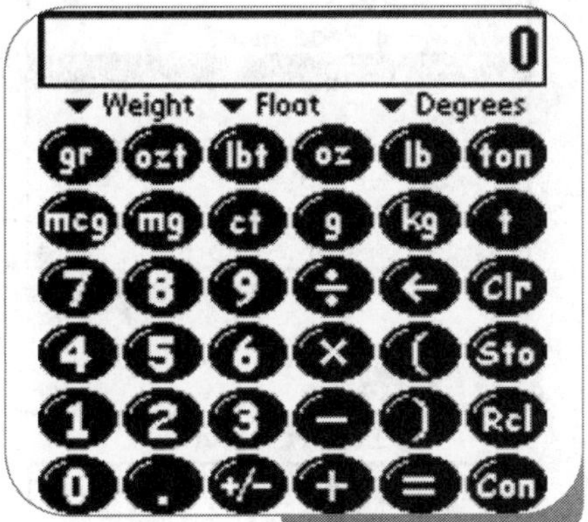

Figure 95A

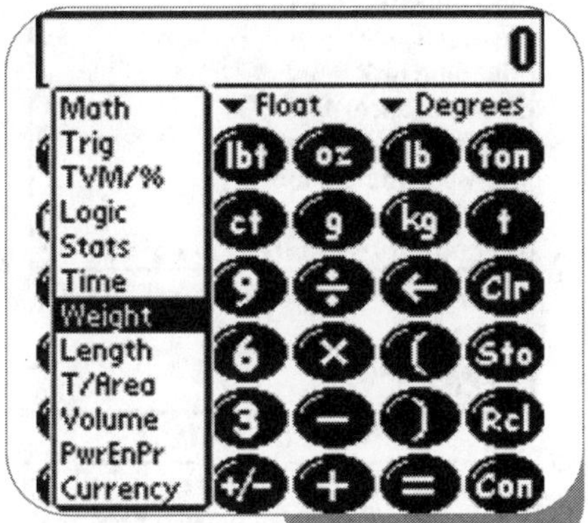

Figure 95B

The other nice thing is that you can reset the button on your PDA to make Parens the default setting for your calculator. Go to Prefs on your PDA launch screen. Tap Buttons in the upper right-hand corner dropdown menu. Tap Calculator and select Parens from the list. You're now all set to have an advanced calculator that is readily available at the touch of a button.

■ MedRules, version 2.5, 2002, by Kent E. Willyard, M.D.

Dr. Willyard has done it again. This is a program that only a medical professional in the trenches could appreciate. Not only does this calculator have 41 unique equations, but also it is user friendly, does the calculation for you automatically, and has references for each equation. What more could you ask for? I purposely omitted the memory requirements for this program because they are variable. MedRules consists of three components, all of which are necessary to run the program properly. You may find that you have already installed one or more of the components to run some other program. In that case, you would not need to install all three again. At most, the installation of all three components would require 324K of memory. This freeware program is worth the small incursion on your PDA's memory. I just want to show you a bit of what it has to offer. First, Figure 96 shows you the four-page menu of equations.

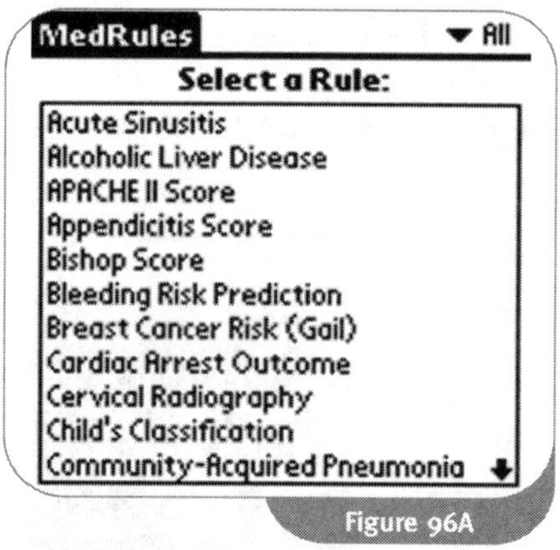
MedRules
All
Select a Rule:
Acute Sinusitis
Alcoholic Liver Disease
APACHE II Score
Appendicitis Score
Bishop Score
Bleeding Risk Prediction
Breast Cancer Risk (Gail)
Cardiac Arrest Outcome
Cervical Radiography
Child's Classification
Community-Acquired Pneumonia
Figure 96A

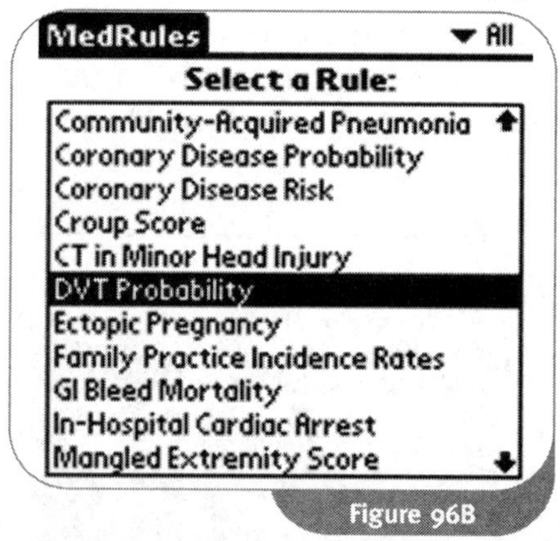

Figure 96B

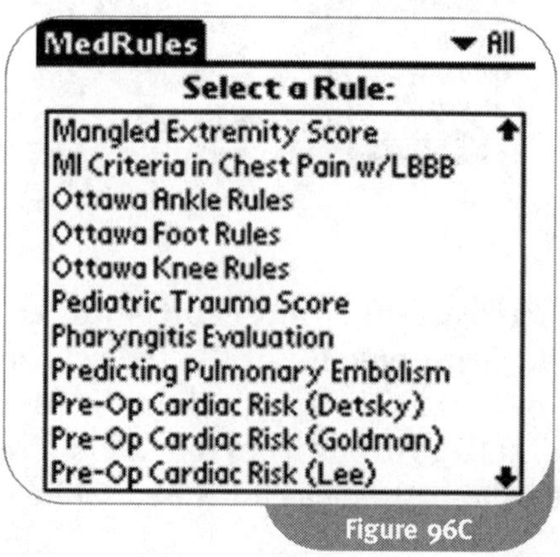

Figure 96C

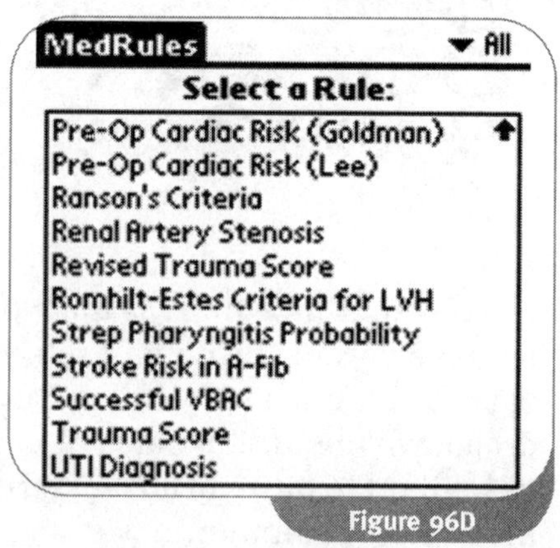

Figure 96D

As you can see, quite a selection is available. Then select one, such as DVT Probability (Figure 96B), from the menu. Figure 97 shows what the DVT calculator looks like.

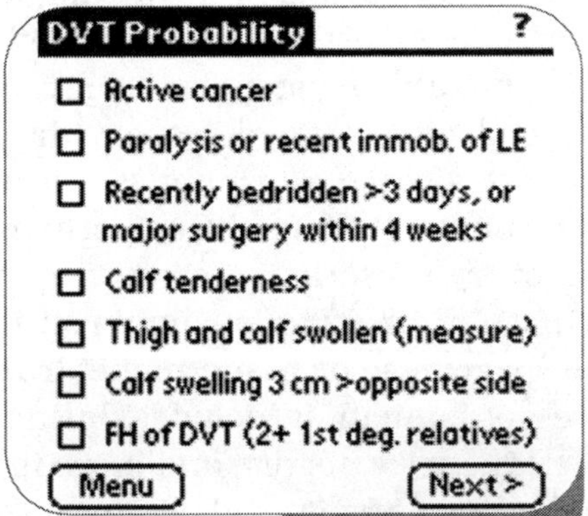

Figure 97A

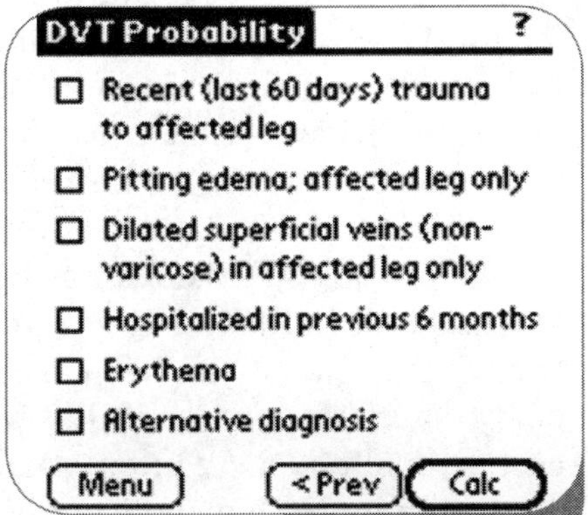

Figure 97B

You can see that this particular equation requires two pages of input; however, they are simple checkboxes, and then the calculator does the math. Tap on the question mark in the upper right-hand corner to get the reference for this particular equation (Figure 98).

The author is quick to point out that this is only for educational purposes and includes the standard disclaimers, but this is a true example of evidence-based medicine at its finest.

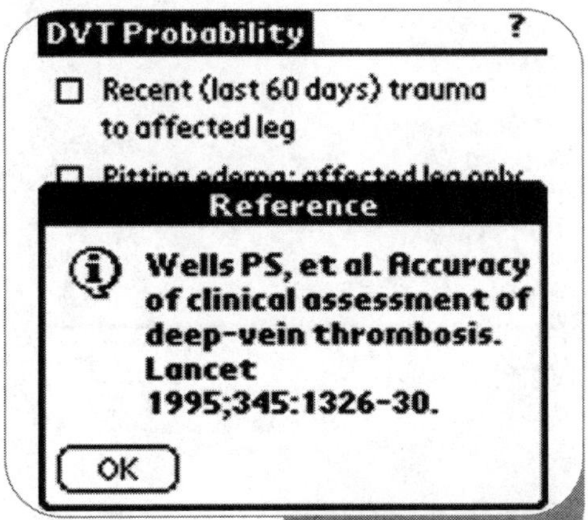

Figure 98

ePocrates qRx

I would be very disappointed and sorry if you did not make it to this point in the book. That's because it has taken me this long to get to one of the most revolutionary programs available in medicine for the PDA. I firmly believe that the single best reason for a medical professional to get and use a handheld computer today is ePocrates (that's what most of us call ePocrates qRx every day) (www.ePocrates.com). The reasons are simple: ePocrates is a free prescription drug database that is updated frequently (perhaps weekly). It probably does not have every prescription drug known to mankind, but it has every one that I'm likely to encounter. It is user friendly, as it can be searched by generic or brand name drug or by drug category. As if that were not enough, it includes dosing, cost, side effect, drug interaction, pregnancy category, and more information on each drug listed. Finally, one version of ePocrates also includes a hidden treasure chest of Regimens and Tables. For example, Figure 99 shows the top of the list, sorted by drug name, updated on April 11, 2001 (I only mention that in case you're wondering where such-and-such new drug is).

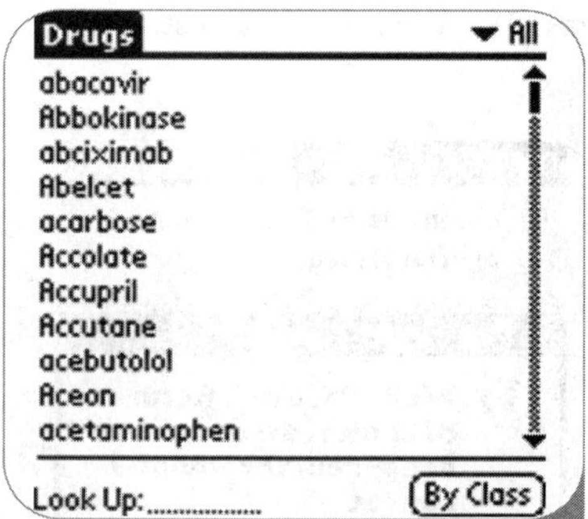

Figure 99

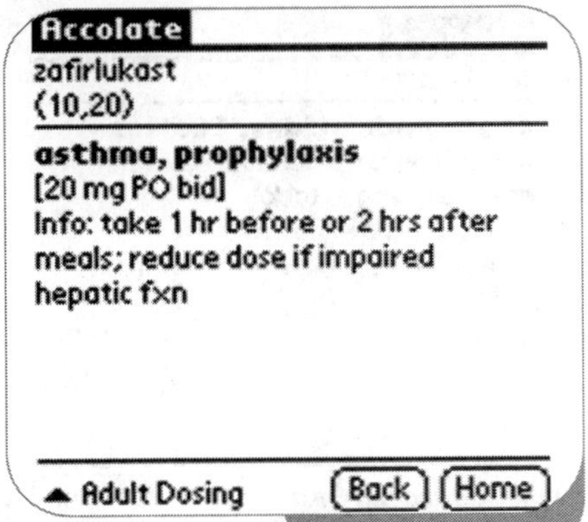

Figure 100

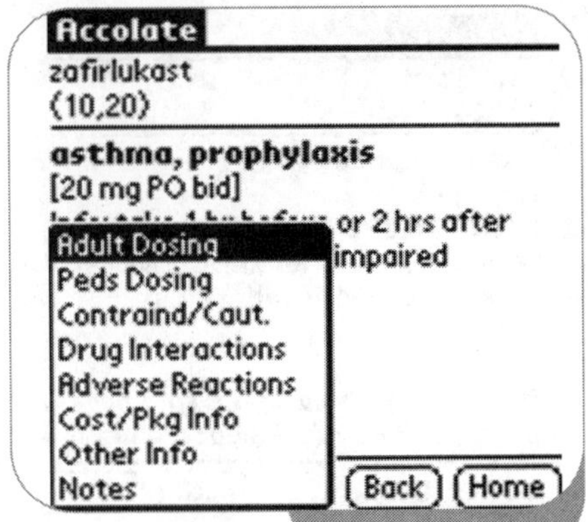

Figure 101

Let's explore what the database has to offer if we tap on Accolate. We'll see the screen shown in Figure 100, which includes generic name, dosage forms available, indications, and adult dosing.

We can also see that there is an arrow next to Adult Dosing, indicating that a popup list is available. If we tap on this, the list shown in Figure 101 will be revealed.

Just for the purposes of illustration, I'll show you each of the screens that would be revealed by tapping on each of the items in the popup list for this one drug, Accolate (Figure 102).

The final item on the popup list, Notes (Figure 101), allows you to make a few of your own notes to attach specifically to this drug. If we tap the Back button, we come back to the original screen of drug listings. Tap By Class in the lower right-hand corner of the screen to see the database sorted by drug categories rather than drug names. In Figure 103, you see this and a second screen shot of what you get if you continue to scroll through the classes. Notice the "Other" category.

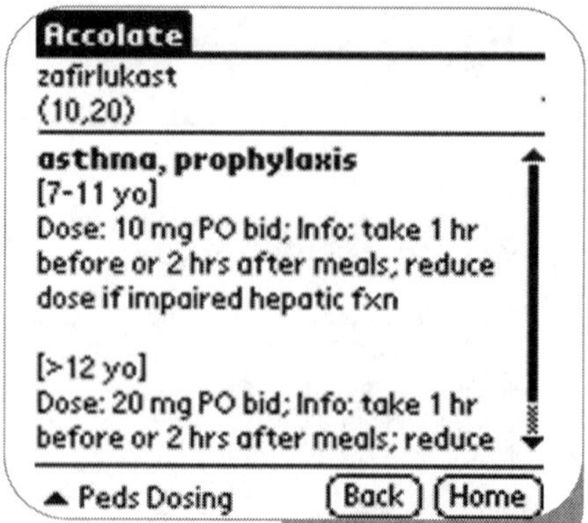

Figure 102A

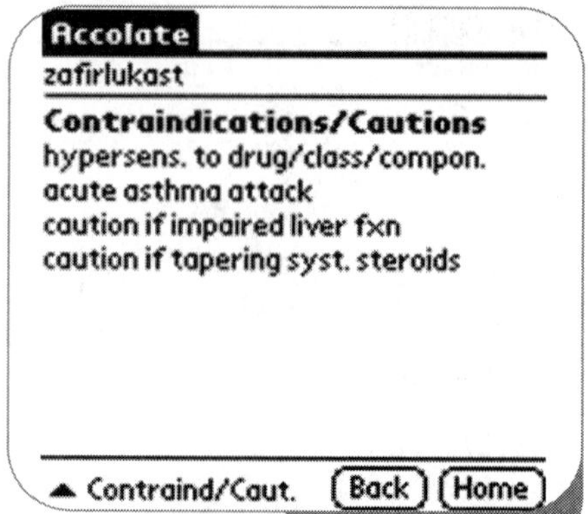

Figure 102B

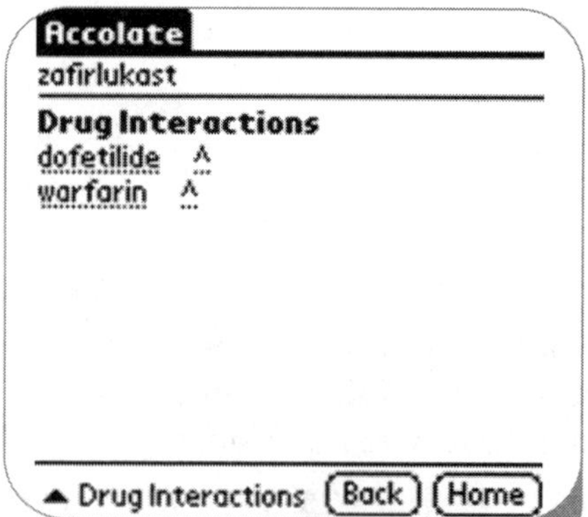

Figure 102C

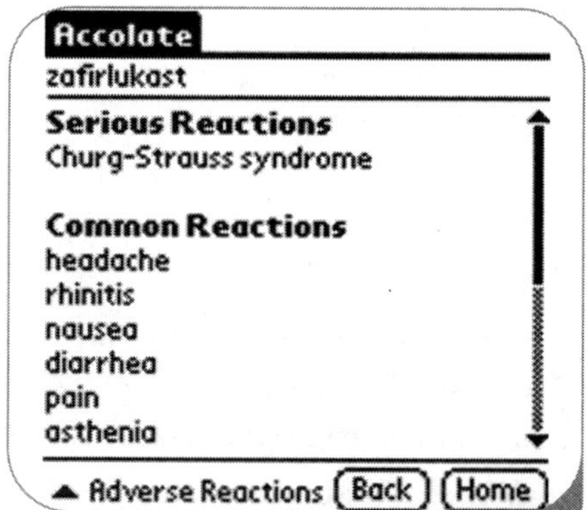

Figure 102D

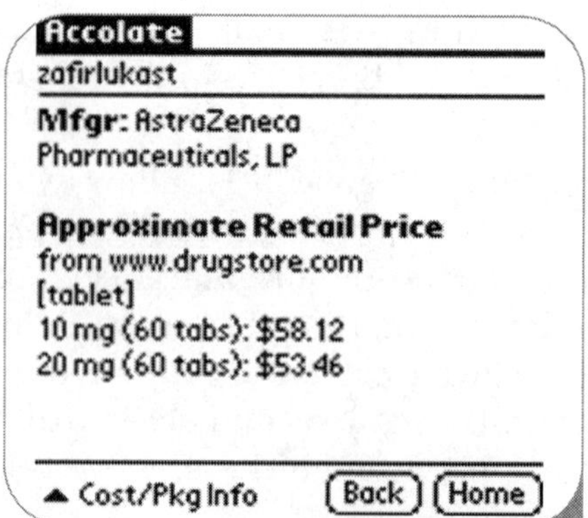

Figure 102E

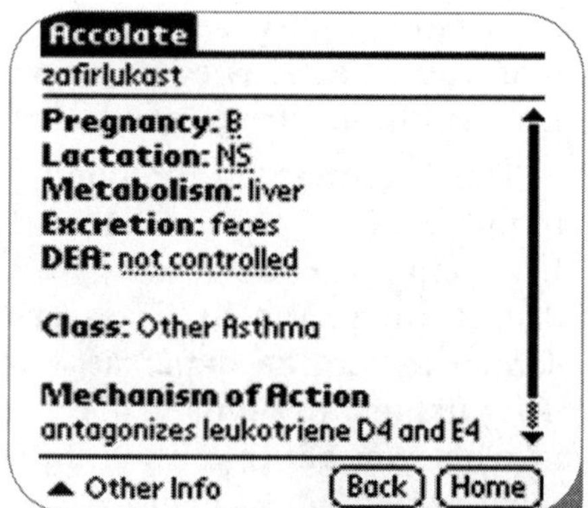

Figure 102F

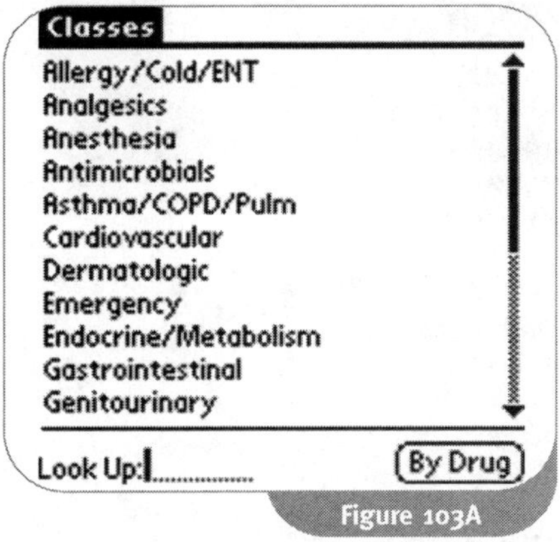

Figure 103A

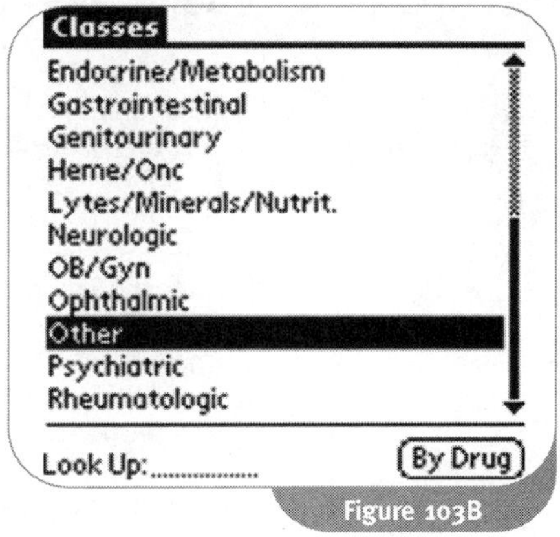

Figure 103B

The Other class (actually accessible also from the Drug list) is the repository of that hidden treasure chest of Regimens and Tables that I referred to previously. This list of Regimens and Tables is available in only the ePocrates Pro version ($49.99 per year currently) (Figure 104). Tap on Regimens and Tables and you will be able to scroll through two pages of the aforementioned.

The value to the practicing clinician of having this information readily available is incalculable. It is also updated constantly. Therefore, you'll have the latest ACLS protocols, American Heart Association guidelines, and narcotic equivalents in your PDA. You'll have the latest vaccination schedule and know what to do when someone misses a dose. You'll have an answer for patients who don't know the name

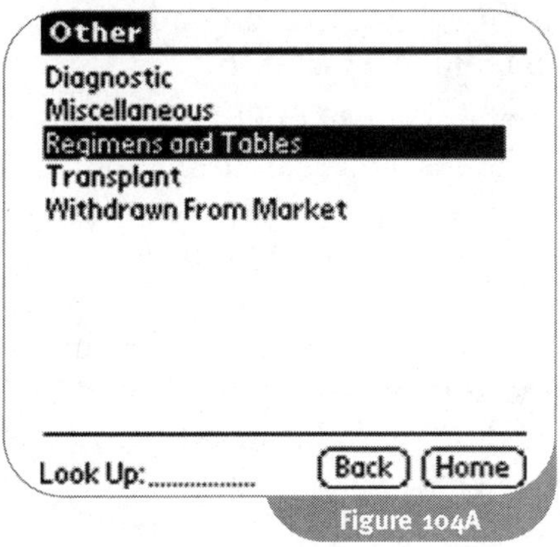

Figure 104A

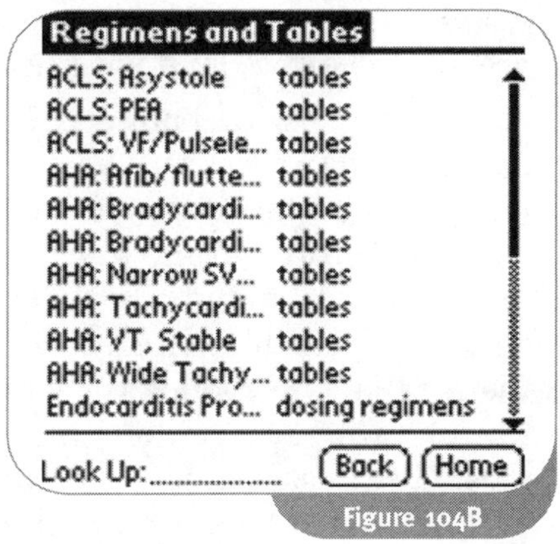

Figure 104B

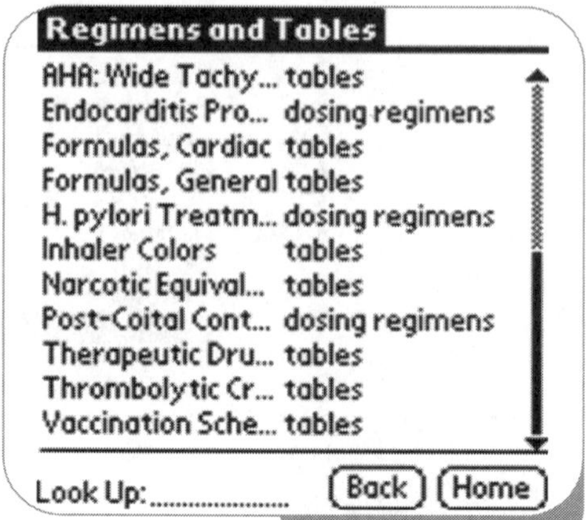
Regimens and Tables
AHA: Wide Tachy... tables
Endocarditis Pro... dosing regimens
Formulas, Cardiac tables
Formulas, General tables
H. pylori Treatm... dosing regimens
Inhaler Colors tables
Narcotic Equival... tables
Post-Coital Cont... dosing regimens
Therapeutic Dru... tables
Thrombolytic Cr... tables
Vaccination Sche... tables
Look Up:
Back
Home
Figure 104C

of the drug in their metered dose inhaler, but you can tell them what it is by the color of the packaging. This feature just fascinates me. The folks at ePocrates have really poured a lot of useful information into their database.

Even more features are available in this incredible database that deserve your time and attention. For example, if you have to deal with one or more approved formularies in your practice, chances are that it can be designated in the formularies section of ePocrates. Then when you want to make a prescribing decision, you will also know whether the drug you want to prescribe is on formulary, whether it is the preferred choice on that particular formulary, etc. This can be quite useful to clinicians who have to deal with HMOs and various types of insurance coverage. Not all local and regional formularies are available yet, but more are being added constantly.

The web site has complete instructions for the entire registration and download process, which I'm afraid is a bit tedious, but not difficult. It is also interesting to note, if you read the fine print, that the download process from ePocrates is a two-way street. You get updated information from them, and they, in turn, get usage pattern information from your handheld during the process. They explain that although that information is never identified with you individually, it is useful in the aggregate to pharmaceutical and marketing companies. This, in part, is how ePocrates is available to us all free. The company recently announced, in the past few months, the 700,000th user of ePocrates.

ePocrates Pro

I won't go into great detail about this latest offering from the ePocrates web site, but it is sufficiently important to deserve further mention. Moreover, I'm including this version here in the freeware/shareware section, even though it is $49.99 per year, because it seems logical to associate it with its free sibling. In practice, ePocrates Pro replaces ePocrates qRx and is really the same database with some extra features built in. Here is the layout with the easy-access tabs (now actually available in both free and Pro versions of ePocrates). The Alternative Meds and Tables are separate tabs and are really available in only the Pro edition. Similarly, the Tool bag is a separate tab and is really available in only the Pro edition. In Figure 105, you see the contents of the Tool bag after you have tapped on it.

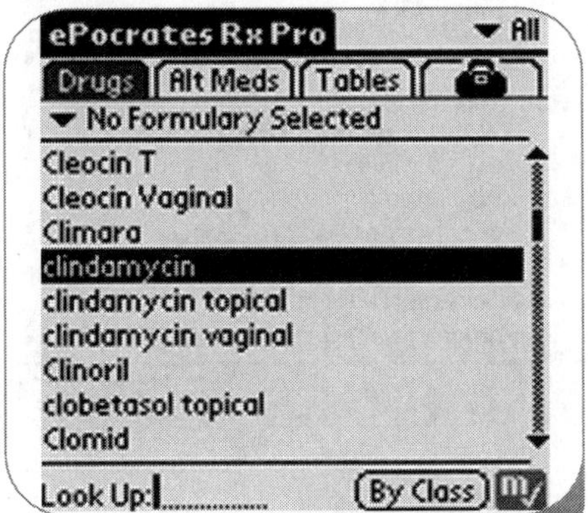

Figure 105A

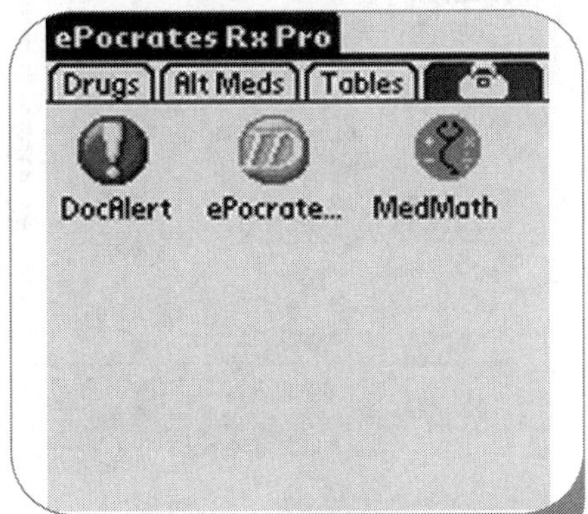

Figure 105B

I have already mentioned the Regimens and Tables feature. ePocrates Pro also includes another amazing feature. It is an infectious disease database that links with the ePocrates database in your handheld. You use this additional ID database to select an empiric drug for a given organism or to indicate empiric treatment for a wide variety of infectious diseases. The database can be searched by location affected, by "Bug" (infectious cause), or by Drug (used to treat) (Figure 106).

You can find out more about this amazing tool at the ePocrates web site. Additionally, the Tool bag contains the latest (2002) version of Phillip Cheng's MedMath, now with 34 equations included. We

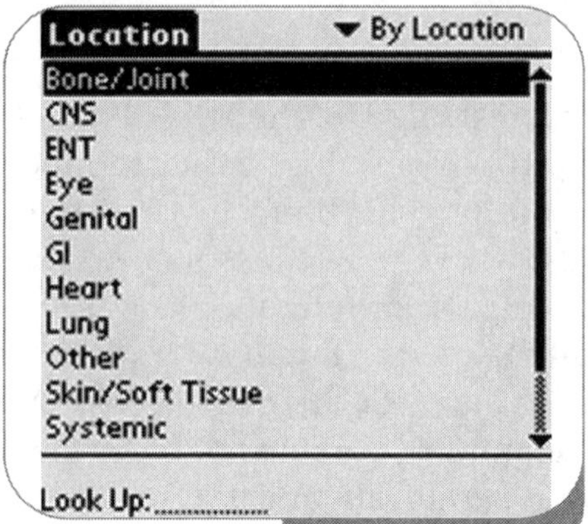

Figure 106A

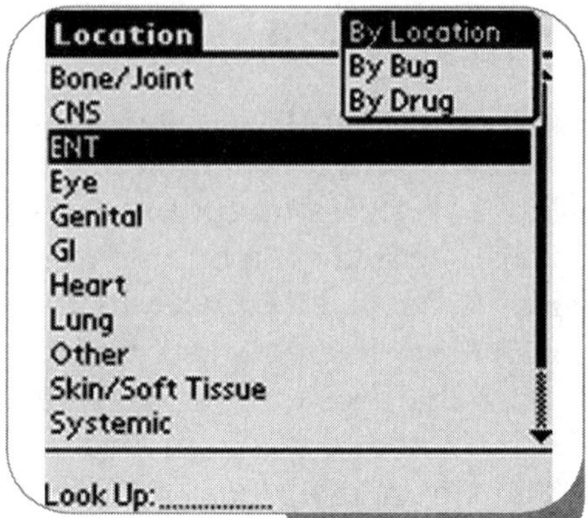

Figure 106B

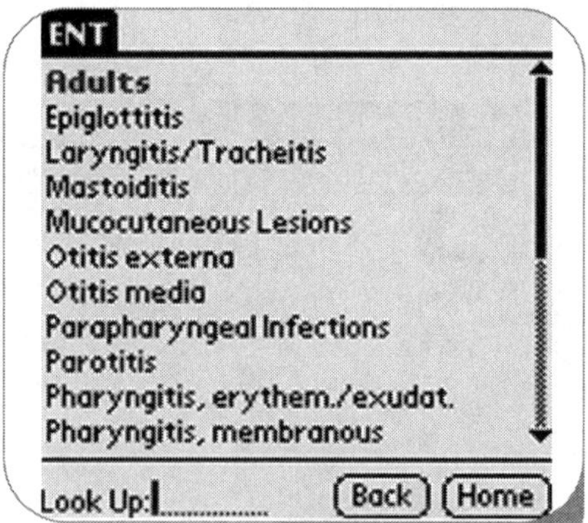

Figure 106C

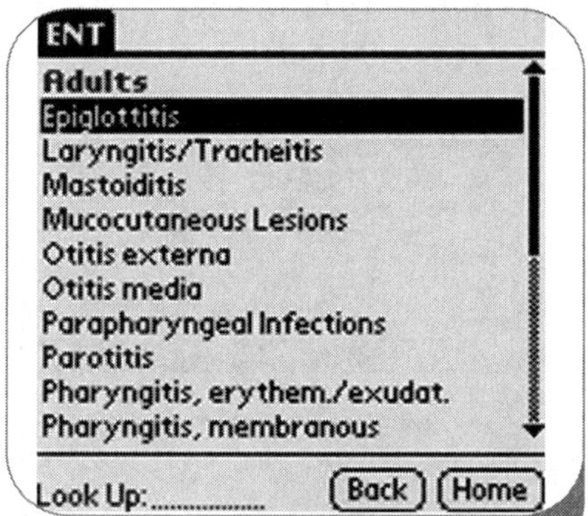

Figure 106D

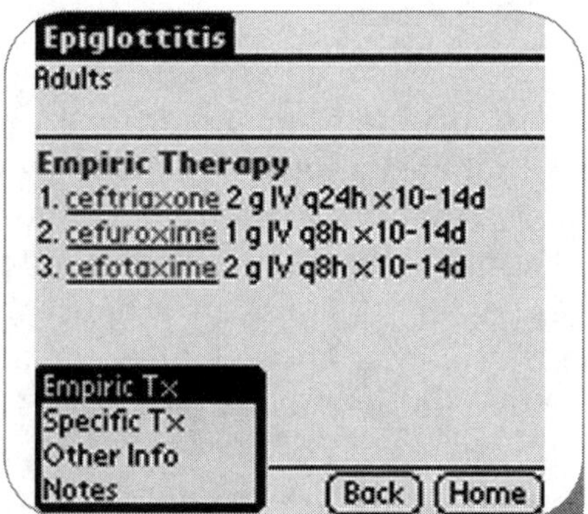

Figure 106E

reviewed this program in Medical Freeware/Shareware, but it is interesting to note that the ePocrates folks thought that it was useful enough to a wide variety of medical professionals that they included it in the Tool bag of ePocrates Pro (Figure 107).

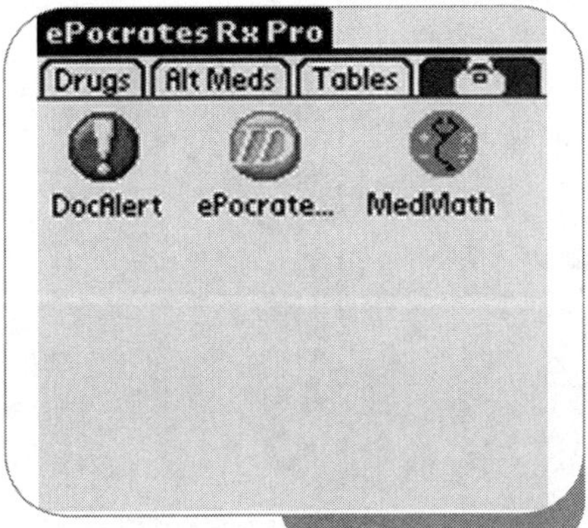

Figure 107A

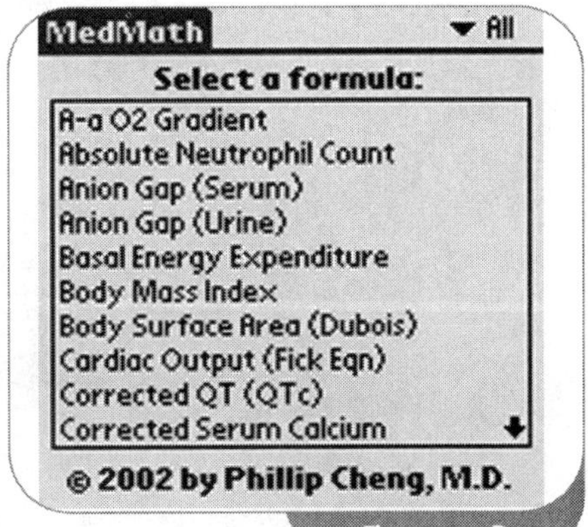

Figure 107B

Mobile PDR

Not to be outdone, the folks at Clinicians Publishing Group who brought you the Physician's Desk Reference (PDR) have also created the Mobile PDR for your handheld (www.pdr.net). It, too, is available free. It was originally available to only full-time practicing clinicians. Recently, however, Mobile PDR has been made available to medical students and residents.

Johns Hopkins University Antibiotic Guide

This database (http://hopkins-abxguide.org/download_center/download_center.cfm) works well for several reasons: ease of use, authority of the source, it is updated periodically, it is free, and it helps to keep competitors honest. First go to the Johns Hopkins University web site and register as a free user, download the database, and install it to your PDA. Unfortunately, this one does not seem to work from external memory. However, you may find it worth having anyway. I can't show you much of the Guide here, but you can see in Figure 108 that it is nicely arranged and simple to use.

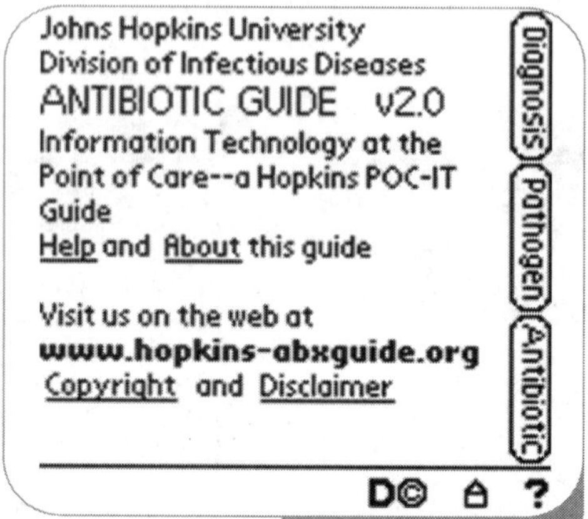

Figure 108

Medical Mnemonics

This wonderful free program (version 2.0.0, 2001, by Adroit Mobile [www.adroitmobile.com]), comes with hundreds of memory aids that we call mnemonics. The database can be sorted or searched by System, Discipline, Knowledge Level, and Body Part. Many useful mnemonics are available here. Because I find the program somewhat hard to navigate, it is a bit hard to use on the fly but great study fodder when you have the time. Authors of the specific items are generally included, although specific literature citations don't appear to exist to support the mnemonics. If you're studying for boards and you like this kind of memory aid, then you'll love this program. Otherwise, it's just fun trivia.

The Prescriber's Letter

This is mentioned because I am a subscriber to the monthly Prescriber's Letter (www.prescribersletter.com), and lately I've noticed that increasingly they are offering free supplements for download to your PDA if you are a subscriber. The last one that I received, which seems very useful, was for common drug interactions with herbal supplements. The Prescriber's Letter now has a number of these Detail Documents that are available on their web site for PDA download. Subscribers can even download the latest edition of the Letter itself to their PDA so that it could be read or referred to later on the go. I believe this sort of offering will be an increasing trend with a number of medical publishers. Publishers are always looking for different ways to attract subscribers. As handhelds become increasingly widespread in the medical field, free and useful PDA downloads will surely be an attractive supplement. Look for more of these.

Tarascon ePharmacopoeia

Many medical professionals are familiar with the tiny pocket-sized print version of this truly handy drug database (version 1.6.04 [1098K of memory], 2002, copyright 2001, by Tarascon Publishing [http://tarasconpublishing.com/store/palm.asp]). I have appreciated my copy during my clinical training. Alas, my eyes aren't what they used to be, and the tiny type still is just as tiny. PDA version to the rescue. This is eminently more useful and readable to me. For an electronic drug database, it's fairly complete and small in memory usage.

The Tarascon ePharmacopoeia has been undergoing some product development lately. I have been testing one of the preproduction releases of Tarascon Deluxe and am excited about the prospect of the final release. The product is user friendly with convenient tabs across the top. These take you to a Class (of drugs) list, an Index list, a drug Interact (ions) list, or a Tools list. With these tabs, you can easily navigate and use a lookup feature at almost any point.

There are 20 major drug classes from which to choose, each conveniently subdivided into a multitude of subclasses, from which a subset of the Drug list will pop up. Alternatively, the user could search the Index directly by scrolling through it, jumping to a specific letter of the alphabet from a pick list, or entering a drug name into the Lookup (search) feature. Drugs are listed by both generic and trade names.

The Tools tab has 52 extremely useful tables in it. These are easily accessed and contain a wealth of clinician-friendly information. The Tools are well thought out and are organized by specialty. Here, for example, you will find the Glasgow Coma Scale under Neurology,

Heparin Dosing under Hematology, Topical Steroids under Dermatology, Opioid Equivalency under Analgesics, Antidotes under Toxicology, and much more. The Tarascon folks have packed quite a compendium into the Tools alone. The database portion of the program is accessible from external memory card, as you would expect from a sizable database. I'm eagerly awaiting the release of the final software. It will be interesting to learn the cost and the frequency of updating the database, but this one should be watched carefully.

InfoRetriever

This is an interesting free program to entice you into the company's other, more complete commercial products (version 4.2 [931K of memory], 2002, by InfoPOEMs [www.infopoems.com]). It is, as the makers indicate, "a subset of the information from the desktop, web, and PocketPC versions of InfoRetriever, with a focus on bedside diagnosis." It's hard for me to imagine how much more complete the paid versions of this product could be. A wealth of information is contained here. For now, unfortunately, InfoRetriever works only from internal memory. Maybe later it will be accessible from external memory cards, thereby freeing up more of your PDA's native memory.

POEM is the company's acronym for Patient-Oriented Evidence that Matters, and it certainly appears that this product has a lot of it. This is evidence-based medicine in action. The user can select from a large number of Clinical Decision Rules, Diagnostic Tests, and History and Physical features, and input their values, and the program will calculate the results. Each test, rule, or exam element has been thoroughly studied, and extensive literature references are given to support the evidence. This is a futuristic decision support tool. The initial screen and just a few of the Decision Rules choices are shown in Figure 109.

By pursuing the Stroke branch of the Decision Rules tree, you can see that the user might select the Ischemic vs. hemorrhagic decision rule. Then you can see a portion of the actual decision calculator to determine the likelihood of a hemorrhagic stroke (Figure 110).

Finally, by tapping on the "?" in the upper right-hand corner, the user is taken to the very thorough reference supporting the decision rules. Figure 111 shows a portion of that supporting evidence regarding this particular decision rule.

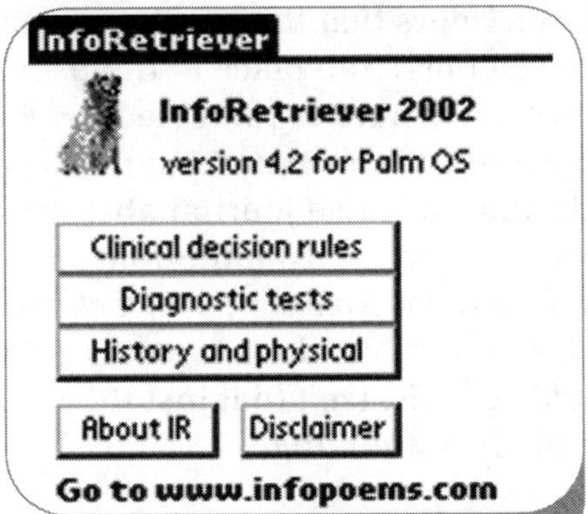

Figure 109A

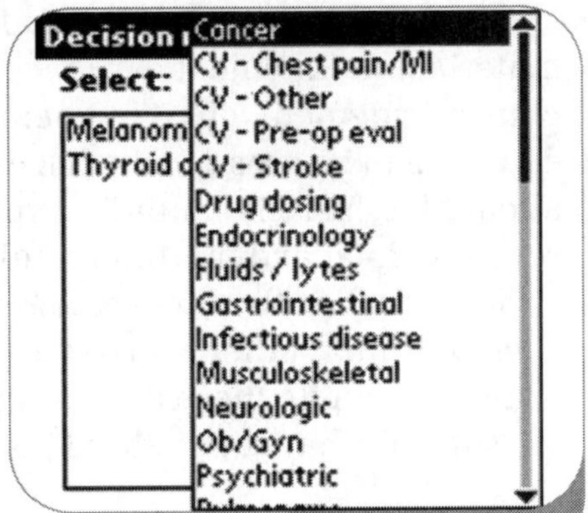

Figure 109B

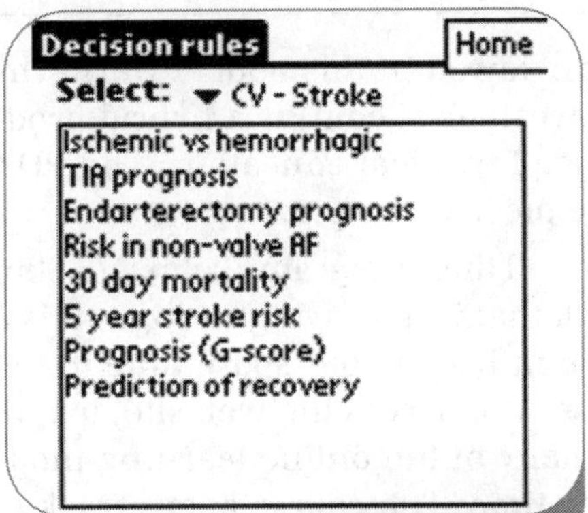

Figure 110A

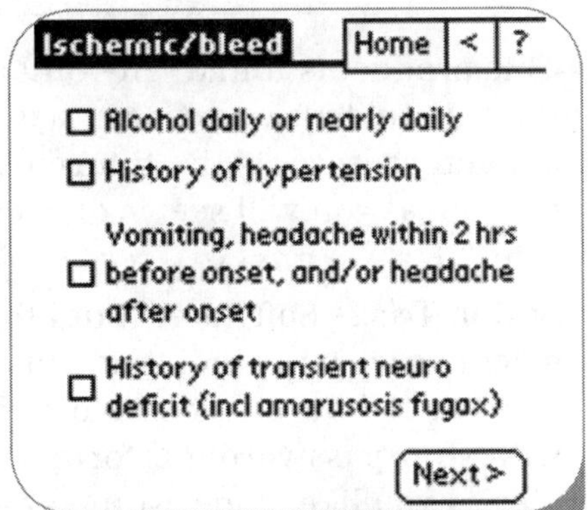

Figure 110B

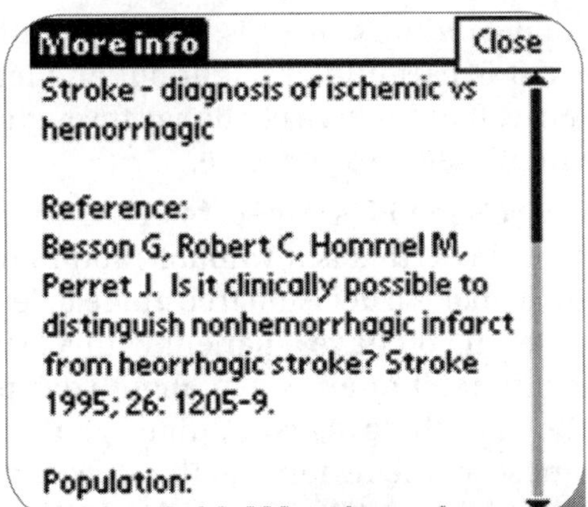

Figure 111

Of course, there are the usual disclaimers that this is educational material, not intended as advice, doesn't take the place of the user's clinical judgment, etc. That being said, it is hard to imagine how we could fail to be greatly aided in our clinical decision making by using a tool like this. The authors explain that they use journal abstracts, reviews, data, and treatment guidelines derived from the *Journal of Family Practice*, the *Evidence-Based Practice* newsletter, the *Cochrane Collaboration*, other journal articles and public domain sources in order to compile these decision making tools. Isn't that just the kind of synthesis that goes behind good medical thinking?

eDerm

This product is unlike any other reviewed in this book. eDerm (by West Portal Software Corp.; www.westportal.com) is a hybrid product and represents the future of good medical education. The PDA portion, as you will see, is only one piece of the pie.

The folks at West Portal Software call their program "Palm O/S Skin Lesion Triage Software," but I think that is not saying enough. It is a teaching/learning tool that you can utilize in your spare time in the comfort of your own home or office. You access the web site, log on with your password, perform as many of the online learning modules as you like, and resume at any time. The course keeps track of your progress and scores your quizzes for you, showing your weaknesses any time that you would like to review.

The content of the online course is first rate. Full of color pictures and case studies, it is carefully thought out and leads to a valuable learning experience. It becomes a challenge throughout to better yourself. It is a true multimedia experience.

To top it off, there's the PDA aspect of eDerm. Occupying just 59K of memory on your PDA, this is a valuable addition to your portable armamentarium. It places a decision tree guide to lesions right in your handheld computer. If you have a patient with a lesion and input parameters one at a time, it queries you about your patient and his or her lesion. In the end, the program guides you to a most complete differential diagnosis of the lesion and the steps that you should take with the patient at this point. The PDA tool is, by itself, worth the price of admission and worthy of your attention.

More information is available through the West Portal web site listed previously. I have recently found the site a bit difficult to navigate, but a contact point for the developers is available for further information on eDerm and their other products. Also, try the alternative site (www.edermpda.com) for a demonstration of the product and other contact points for the developers. When it comes to derm lesions, whether you think you know it all or whether you think you've forgotten it all, this site deserves attention. I would like to see West Portal apply this type of beautifully integrated learning to other medical specialties.

BioChem/BioChem 1st RespondER

This is really two different programs of identification and action to be taken for biochemical terrorist attacks (Arkansoft software; http://www.geocities.com/arkansoft). The first is the Freeware version, the lay product, BioChem. The second is the commercial product, BioChem 1st RespondER (free trial version, $14.95 for the full registered version), made for professionals in the field. You can immediately sense the timeliness of these products. The information is based on data from the U.S. Centers for Disease Control.

The two products are organized the same way, but the professional version is more complete in its listings and includes more action tabs. Both versions are organized around (1) chemical agents, (2) biological agents, and (3) nerve agents with tabs that guide the user to "find name of agent based on . . ." appearance or odor. Based on these action tabs, the full version has 16 Chemical Agents from Chloropiricin to White Phosphorous, 9 Biological Agents from Anthrax to Tularemia, and 4 Nerve Agents (Sarin, Soman, Tabun, and VX). Furthermore, Appearance lists 11 choices based on color and oiliness and Odor lists 14 choices. All products and all choices are not available in the freeware lay version.

Once you choose an agent, you can seek further information under these headings: Symptoms, Odor, Appearance, 1st Aid, Delivery Method, and Cautions. The 1st RespondER version then adds four more tabs: 1st Meds, ER Care, ER Meds, and Lab. As stated in the product, these are to add "treatments, drugs, and dosages to administer, both at the disaster site and afterward in the hospital, as well as lab tests to order and advanced data on patient care."

These are well thought-out guides, user friendly for rapid access, and very timely in their subject matter. Hopefully, none of us will ever need to make use of such a reference, but it's good to know that it exists. If I were working in the field of Emergency Medicine, I would especially want to be armed with such a reference.

Acupressure and Do-in

The software author Fernando Villanova also has several other programs available at the web site (www.acheishopping.com.br/villanova), version 2.0, April 2002, by Kevin T. Boyd. A few of these are shareware, but most of them are freeware (check out his freeware First Aid program, too).

I was never taught, nor do I pretend to understand, this alternative medicine therapy. Nonetheless, some of our patients will undoubtedly be coming in with questions regarding this type of modality. It certainly can't hurt to have a reference like this available, and the price is a bonus. The program is small, well organized, and has elegantly simple illustrations. Do-in (as it's called in its icon) takes up very little space for an illustrated program. The .PRC file is only 168K, and the .PDB file is less than 14K. You would also need to install the current version of NSB Runtime (approximately 90K).

Once you have tapped the Do-in icon, the program takes a couple of seconds to load to your PDA (since I store mine in an external memory card) (Figure 112).

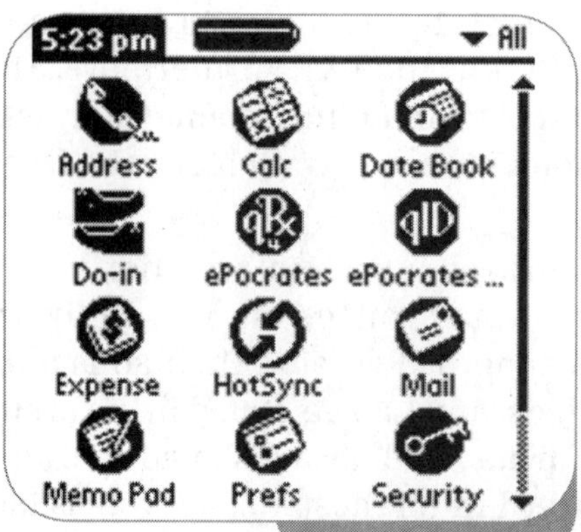

Figure 112A

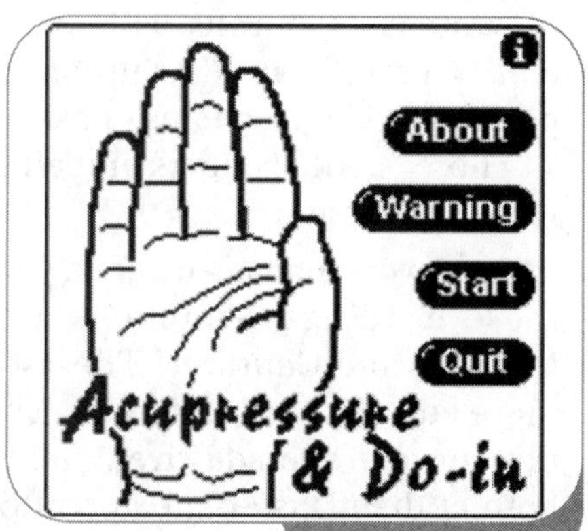

Figure 112B

You then select the Body Area from Head, Trunk, Limbs, or Body/Anywhere. Then you select Symptom/pain location from a drop-down menu. This takes you to a specific Acupoint (or points) with a figure and description of each point (Figure 113).

This is a fun piece of software. It shows off the illustrative power of your PDA and does it at a price that everyone can afford (free).

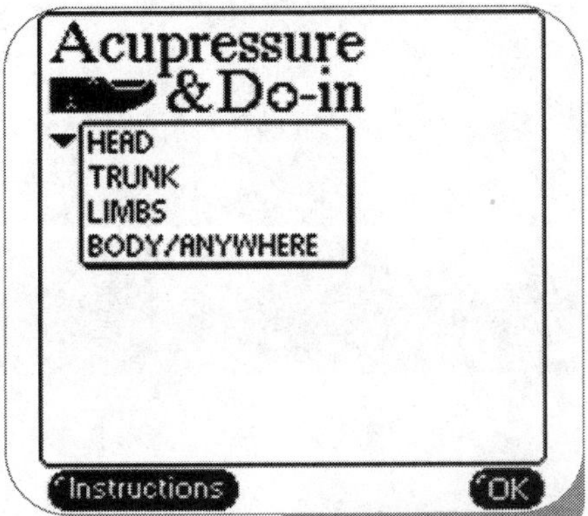

Figure 113A

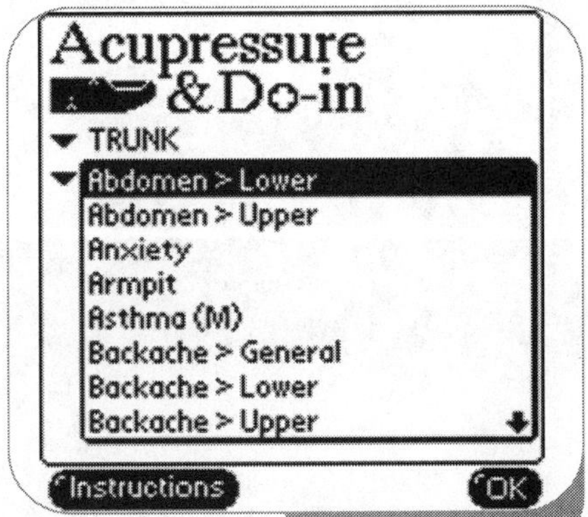

Figure 113B

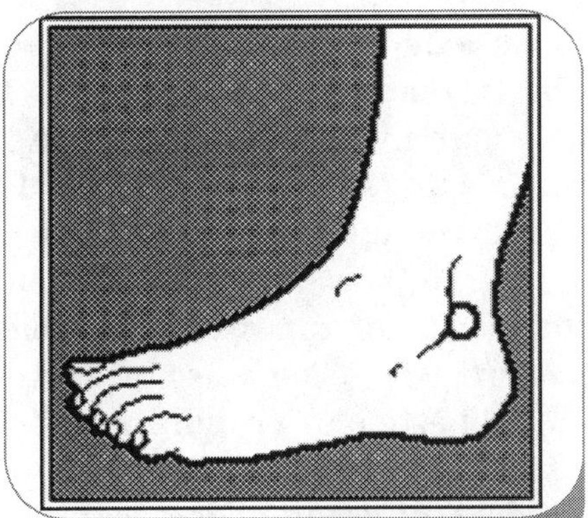

Figure 113C

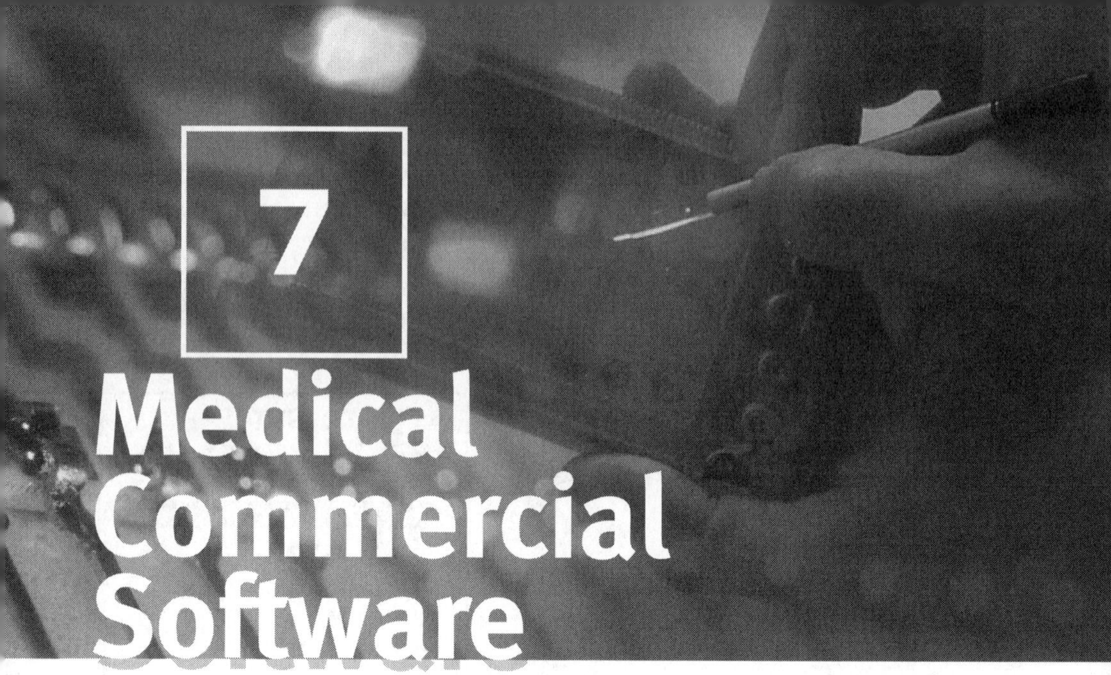

7 Medical Commercial Software

Texts: Skyscape and Others

Probably one of the greatest areas of growth in medical commercial software for the PDA is that of e-books, or texts. Why shouldn't it be? Texts in your handheld computer seem natural. Not only can you carry a lot of information in a tiny space, but you can also access it anytime and anywhere and search it more quickly than the printed version. Here is just a representative sample of medically useful titles with which I am familiar, although many are available. You may find that you like features of one type of software over another and thus want to concentrate on that particular brand. You should also know if that occurs, some titles are available in more than one software brand. For the most up-to-date information, you are referred to the applicable web site.

Washington Manual of Medical Therapeutics

This venerable and respected clinical reference has been around in the print version since 1943. The PDA version is a natural of portability with an ease of use that is common to the Skyscape products.

A tap on the product icon on the handheld launch screen takes you immediately into *The Washington Manual* (30th edition, powered by Skyscape, version 4.0.32, $59.95), where the first screen reveals the "Wash Mnl" name in the upper left-hand corner and below that a drop-down arrow with three choices: Main Index, Medication Index, or Table of Contents. Thoughtfully, each of these are further explained by a tap of the "i" (or information) icon near the top right corner. The visual orientation of the Table of Contents usually makes it a logical choice for me.

A tap on the Table of Contents reveals 26 chapters and 8 appendices. A perusal of chapter headings will look familiar to anyone familiar with the print version of *The Washington Manual.* The variety of the chapter headings seems fairly comprehensive to me. I also like the appendices that follow, especially the laboratory reference values.

Each of the chapters and appendices, in turn, displays the now familiar "+" sign to its left. A tap of the "+" expands to display the contents of the requested chapter. For example, tap the "+" next to Chapter 4, Hypertension, to reveal that this chapter includes articles on "Definitions and Diagnostic Evaluation, Therapeutic Considerations, Special Considerations and Tables." In turn, tap the "+" next to Tables to reveal that the chapter includes tables on manifestations of target organ disease, classification of blood pressure for adults age 18 years and older, commonly used antihypertensive agents by functional class, and intravenous antihypertensive drug preparations. Where any chapter or table title is too long to fit on one line of the screen, a small arrow to the right, when tapped, reveals the rest of the title briefly. The list of tables or the list of articles within the chapter can be compressed again by tapping the now present "–" sign next to the heading. The exploded view is now compressed again and the familiar "+" sign is back in its place. I like this system and feel that it should become the standard.

If a Table of Contents search is not to your liking, tap the drop-down arrow next to Table of Contents, select Main Index, and peruse *The Washington Manual* by index item. This offers the added advantage of being able to scrawl a search word in the bottom "Look for: ______" area of the screen. When I scribbled "hypertension" in here using Graffiti, I was brought to the area of the index with all of the items that start with "hypertension." Tap on this particular entry of the index and the various chapter headings of Chapter 4, Hypertension are revealed. If, however, you were to select a more specific index listing, such as "hypertensive emergency," a Topic Outline would be shown that could very quickly take the user to more specific information details. Tap the "M" icon in the upper right corner to return immediately to the Main Index to reselect from the index.

Alternatively, you could select Medication Index from the dropdown arrow at top left. Using Graffiti in the "Look for: _______" area, we might write "at" and be immediately drawn to the entry for "Atenolol." Tap on this entry and you'll be shown an array of entries that can be selected for further clarification on this particular drug regarding such topics as "Overdosage, Stable Angina, Therapeutic Considerations," and more. Select any one of these of interest to once again be brought to an expanded screen, including a Topic Outline and articles delineated under sections. An added feature that is available on some of these expanded views is an icon resembling an eye. Tap on this eye icon to go instantly to an array of related topics, from which you are easily able to return to the previous topic or move on to the next topic.

Getting used to the controls and icons takes only a few minutes and is well worth the time spent. The Skyscape folks have broken a book down into small, easily accessible increments that are easy to search and easy to reference. The alternative of reading endless text would be okay for the library, but not for the bedside. The system is user friendly and intuitive. Once mastered, you could use it on most any of the other 100-odd Skyscape products as well.

An added bonus is that *The Washington Manual*, as other Skyscape products, works quite well from external memory. This is important to know since you have only limited internal memory on your PDA. The major memory hogs of these e-books are the .pdb (database) files. These can be safely installed to external memory so that a number of e-books can be contained on a single external memory card. Only the .prc (program) files, which are much smaller, need to be installed in your PDA's internal memory.

Washington University Internship Survival Guide

This medical PDA reference is great for its punchy, bulleted style. It doesn't try to be a library. It hits the high points, the real keys to student survival, and also includes sufficient detail and information to make intelligent decisions. Finally, it is easily navigable. What good is the best information if you can't find it?

The key to the navigation of *The Washington University Internship Survival Guide* (hereafter, WUINSurv; powered by Skyscape $29.95) is the now legendary Skyscape software platform. A few minutes spent learning the remarkable features of Skyscape will reward you with speedy and intuitive navigation. Skyscape powers more than 100 mobile medical references; thus, you will master more than WUINSurv at the same time. What's more, if you install more than one Skyscape product to your handheld computer, they automatically cross-link and cross-reference when applicable. This could be invaluable, for example, when you want more extensive or in-depth drug information and your WUINSurv links to one of the Skyscape drug guides.

To review, if you are not familiar with the Skyscape system, three major ways to navigate the text are available. You can surf (1) the Main Index, (2) the Medication Index, or (3) the Table of Contents. In addition, it's important to note that all three of these choices also feature the convenient "Look for ______," which is at the bottom of the page, for the instant gratification that only a "find" feature can provide.

Common to all three navigation modes are Skyscape's patented SmARTbuttons at the top right of each page. SmARTbuttons are graphic buttons that the user taps to link to other Skyscape products, visit recently viewed topics, see index terms, access annotation, or See Also" (related topics) lists. I especially like this last item to follow a logical thread of information in which I might also be interested. In case the user needs help with these various tools (or remembering which is which), helpful instructions are available as a dropdown with each view.

My personal favorite among the three major navigation modes is usually the table of contents mode. I think that this is because I am visually oriented and the table of contents is easy to "drill down" in a graphic outline manner. The table of contents is a masterpiece of organization. WUINSurv is divided into 16 great chapters, the first of which is "Surviving Internship." Tap on its "+" sign to reveal 14 topics within, which include such vital areas as Triage, Admissions, Discharges, and Words to the Wise and Sleep Deprived. Advice is sound, pithy, and bulleted. Just to take the edge off, each topic includes a humorous subtitle. For example, Death/Expirations is subtitled "The celestial discharge."

Of the 16 extremely useful chapters of WUINSurv, I believe that the first five are crucial to the medical student. These are the aforementioned Surviving Internship and four others: Essential Tools, Top Ten Workups, Common Calls and Complaints, and Therapeutics. All of the essentials are here. Then WUINSurv does the amazing. The next nine chapters cover nine specialty areas and their essential consults. These areas range from medicine to dermatology to neurology to general surgery. These well-informed chapters hit the pertinent points of what to look for in each of these specialty areas and what the consultant would be looking for. These points seem extremely useful to me from both the viewpoint of the student and the consultant.

Finally, the last two chapters are Procedures and Critical Care. The former includes concise, step-by-step instructions for performing 11 common invasive procedures (such as phlebotomy, lumbar puncture, and paracentesis), as well as indications, contraindications, equipment, what to tell the patient, complications, and more. The Critical Care chapter includes Cardiac Parameters, Total Parenteral nutrition, Ventilators, and more.

Alternatively, of course, you could navigate WUINSurv via the Main Index or Medication Index modes. Sometimes you will find these search modes to be faster. As with other Skyscape products, WUINSurv works well from external memory. Again, the bulky .pdb (database) file is stored in external memory, and the small .prc (program) file is stored in your PDA's internal memory.

Merck Manual

Over the years, the *Merck Manual* (Centennial edition [17th], by HandHeldMed, 4420K, $79.95) has earned its place as the kind of medical reference that I could quickly turn to when the relatives called for those inevitable free phone consults. I have used the *Merck Manual* print edition extensively, both in my training and in clinical practice. I think that the very simplicity of the *Merck Manual* has often been overlooked in recommending more esoteric, cumbersome, and expensive texts. I have generally turned to the *Merck* first and followed with further reading, if necessary, in those other tomes.

A handheld version would have to be comparable in content, easy to use, and portable. If all that were truly accomplished, then I think one could justify the $79.95 price tag.

At nearly 4.5 MB of memory, the *Merck Manual* is quite a memory hog. It likely couldn't be done with any less memory and still maintain the same thorough content. Mercifully, the *Merck Manual* works just fine from external memory card, as do the other HandHeldMed PDA references. Furthermore, learn the controls of one HandHeldMed product and you have mastered the controls of all of them.

You access the *Merck Manual*, like any other HandHeldMed product, through the HandHeldMed Reader icon on your PDA's launch menu. The Reader is a free download with the purchase of any HandHeldMed product. Tap on the Reader icon and you will be presented with a list of HandHeldMed texts that you have installed to your PDA. In this case, we tap on the *Merck Manual* choice. This opens up the index of the *Merck Manual* that you can scroll or search easily. You can also use the lookup feature to jump to a letter or topic or use the alphabet tabs at the left of the index to jump to a letter in the index, which is all quite quick.

To describe it takes longer than to do it, but I'd like to run through the other navigation features that come into play when you tap on the Reader's right-hand corner dropdown arrow. These are common to all of the HandHeldMed texts. There are 10 navigation features:

1. The Read icon returns the user to the text that was being read, hiding the dropdown box.
2. The Copy Mode allows the user to select paragraphs to copy to the clipboard, presumably for later insertion into documents or for printing.
3. The Add Bookmark feature allows the user to insert electronic bookmarks in order to access frequently used spots in the text rapidly.
4. The Bookmarks feature allows the user to access those bookmarks set in the previously mentioned feature.
5. Search is a feature that allows the user to search for a specific word in the text. You can search either the entire book or "From Here" if you want to go on from the current point in the text. For the word "copper," for example, the search engine locates the first mention of the

word "copper" in the text and also enables you to jump to the next instance of the word "copper" and so on.

6. Preferences is pretty simple, merely allowing the user to choose whether arrow keys will advance the user one line or one page at a time.

7. Contents displays the Table of Contents, which is my favorite feature. This visually lays out the entire outline of the book. You will see listed the introduction and 23 sections. We will explore the sections more closely later. Meanwhile, I want to point out two items in the introduction. Tap on the "+" sign to the left of introduction to open up and reveal several items in the introduction. Being the nerd that I am, I thought "A Centennial History" was a fun 10-minute read about the history of the *Merck Manual* over the past 100 years. If you do not share my curiosity about history, then you can skip this, but just remember that it's there for future reference. Another item in the introduction, however, is the "Guide for Readers," which is a must-read. It takes only a couple of minutes, but you will understand its usefulness immediately. My only regret about the Contents mode is that the *Merck Manual* apparently does not open to this feature automatically (if somebody figures out how to make this a preference setting, please let me know).

8. Index is the mode that we've already explored, the one with which the *Merck Manual* opens.

9. Help is another choice from the dropdown menu. This is another must-read and briefly describes the various navigation tools and features of the program.

10. Exit is the last choice and is the means of exiting one HandHeldMed Reader text (such as *Merck*) and accessing another.

In all, navigation is simple and intuitive, especially for such a large text. Again, the bonus is that learning to navigate one HHM Reader text enables you to master them all.

If you are familiar with the print edition, then you already know the usefulness of the *Merck Manual*. Look at the Table of Contents. Recall that there are 23 sections besides the introduction. Some of these are Nutrition, Gastrointestinal, Pulmonary Disorders, ENT Disorders, Dermatologic Disorders, Neurologic Disorders, Psychiatric Disorders, etc., covering every major system and most any disease entity. Sections on Special Subjects, Clinical Pharmacology, and Poisoning also exist. If you want it at your fingertips, it's here. The depth of the content included is amazing. For example, under Section 23, Poisoning, you will find Chapter 307, Poisoning (which includes articles on Poisoning, Elimination of Poisons, and Specific Poisons), and Chapter 308, Bites and Stings (which includes articles on venomous snakes, venomous lizards, spiders, bees, other biting arthropods, centipedes/millipedes, scorpions, and marine animals). That is thorough! The Special Subjects section, for example, includes chapters on sarcoidosis, smoking cessation, hyperbaric oxygen therapy, geriatric medicine, and more for a total of 12 chapters. The only caveat here is to spend a few minutes browsing these contents every once in awhile just to refresh your memory of the wealth of subjects that are included in Merck.

In a nutshell, I think that the *Merck Manual* is a great tool for practicing clinicians and students of medicine to have at the ready. It's worth the $79.95 price of admission. One could only hope that in the future it could become as affordable as the print version.

Harrison's Principles of Internal Medicine Companion Book

"*Harrison's*" (14th edition, 1998, by McGraw-Hill/Handheldmed [962K]), as most folks in medicine know it, has become a trusted reference and is often used as the main text in many internal medicine courses. This is the companion handbook, a favorite pocket bulger of many medical students. All of the main entries of the larger *Harrison's* are here, without the bulk of the full articles. If you want to read more, go to your larger *Harrison's* on the bookshelf. Convenience and portability are the key words in this case.

As with other Handheldmed titles, you access *Harrison's* from the Handheldmed Reader icon. *Harrison's* has the same easy navigability as other HHM titles. It is divided into an introduction and 16 chapters that are organized by specialties. Chapters include Dermatology, Nutrition, Infectious Diseases, Cardiovascular Diseases, Neurology, Psyc [sic] Disorders, and more. Chapters are further broken down into a multitude of more specific articles. The chapter Respiratory

Diseases, for example, includes 11 separate articles covering subjects from respiratory function through asthma/pneumonitis to thromboembolism and more. *Harrison's* is a very thorough text for its less than 1MB memory requirement.

Of course, as with other HHM texts, *Harrison's* can be easily searched using the search feature, rather than using the table of contents as a lookup. You can easily set bookmarks too for returning to frequently referenced material. In all, *Harrison's* is a valued tool that has earned a place on many clinicians' PDAs.

5 Minute Series

A number of texts in this series exist. You may be familiar with the print titles like *5 Minute Clinical Consult*, *5 Minute Pediatric Consult*, *5 Minute Orthopedic Consult*, and so forth; these are now available for your PDA. They are powered by Skyscape. Similar to the other titles, once you have learned the format, you can easily navigate any of the other texts. Figure 114 shows a page from the index and a sample entry. Other pages pertaining to the topic of Abortion, spontaneous, are easily accessed by the right-hand side toolbar.

These screen shots show that the toolbar conveniently steers you to Basics, Diagnosis, Treatment, Medications, Followup, and Miscellaneous for any topic when they are applicable. These pages are taken from the demo version of *5 Minute Clinical Consult* powered by Skyscape and are used with permission from Skyscape. The full version covers still more topics, does it fully, and stays easy to navigate.

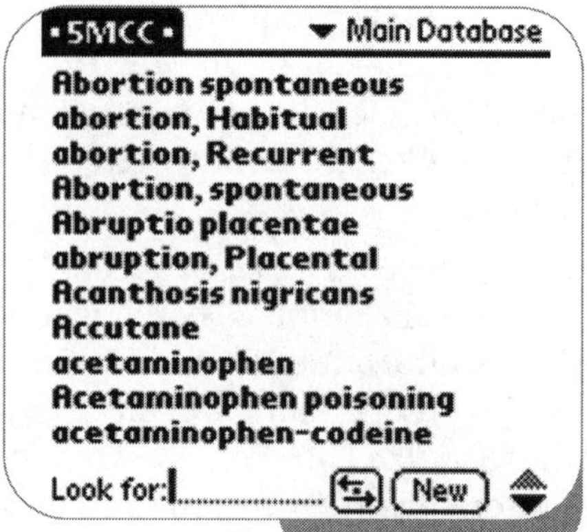

Figure 114A

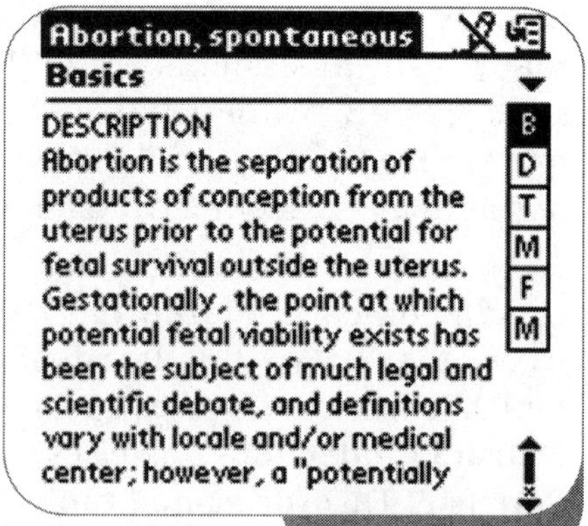

Figure 114B

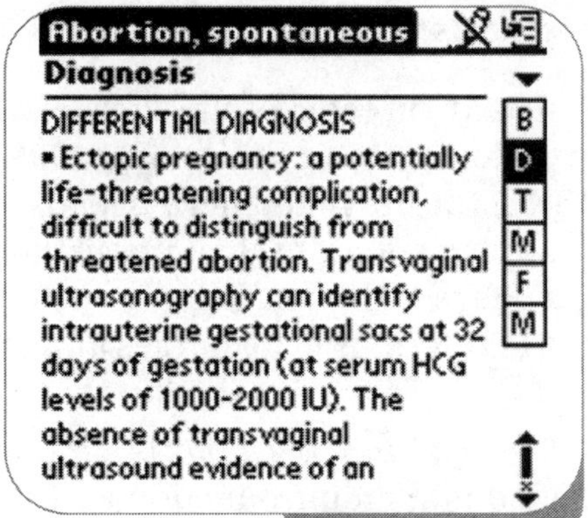

Figure 114C

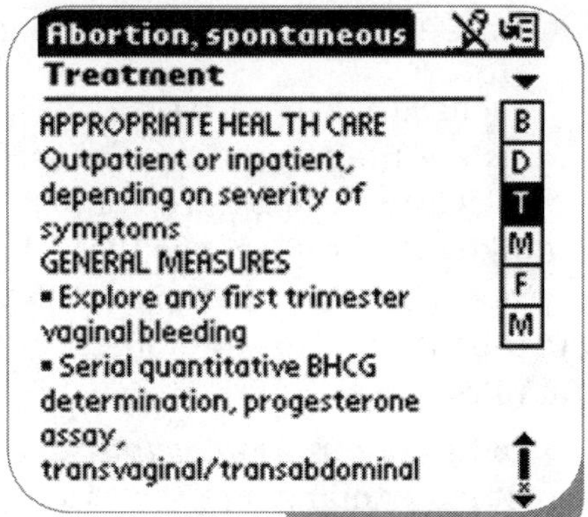

Figure 114D

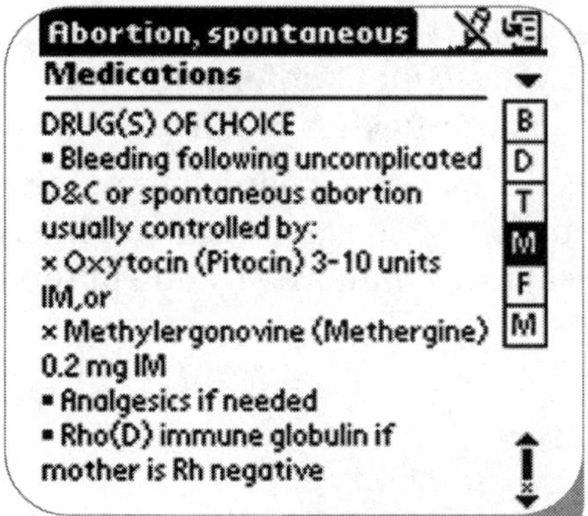

Figure 114E

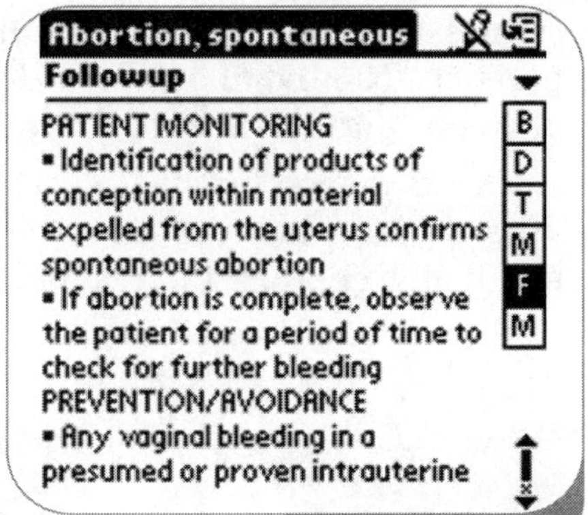

Figure 114F

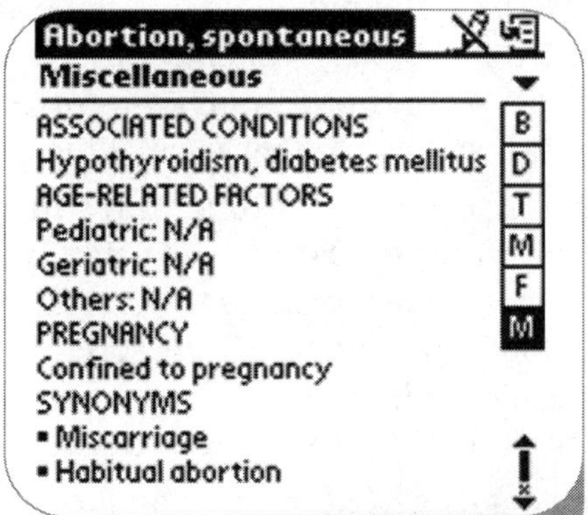

Figure 114G

Moser's Primary Care for Physician Assistants Companion Book

Richard W. Dehn, MPA, PA-C, Assistant Director of the Physician Assistant Program at the University of Iowa, wrote this book (1999, by McGraw-Hill/Handheldmed [618K]). It is included here because, unlike other references that I have reviewed, a physician assistant wrote it for other physician assistants. More of this might be expected in the future, and I anticipate more PDA offerings from nurses aimed at nurses as well.

In its organization, *Primary Care for Physician Assistants* is similar to other primary care texts. It is divided into an introduction and 18 chapters that are organized by specialty. As stated in the preface, the purpose of the handbook is to provide a synopsis of the chapters in the main text. These comprise the diseases and illnesses that a physician assistant is likely to encounter in his or her training or clinical practice. The handbook provides concise, quick information while giving page references to the main text for further reading.

This is a good text that deserves a look by any clinician, not just physician assistants. At the same time, physician assistants will likely find it of even more interest because it was authored by one of their own.

MGH Guide to Psychiatry in Primary Care

Massachusetts General Hospital has had a long and illustrious history in the diagnosis and treatment of psychiatric illnesses. This text (1998, by McGraw-Hill/Handheldmed [679K]) builds on that history and is compiled and edited by a distinguished and experienced panel of clinicians, educators, and reviewers. Each chapter was reportedly coauthored or reviewed by a nonpsychiatrist in order to keep the text relevant and easy-to-use for primary care clinicians.

MGH Psychiatry is organized into an introduction and an unbelievable 78 chapters. Although I enjoy perusing the table of contents, this number of chapters is more likely to compel the user to go to the search function to look up a specific illness. Nearly every psychiatric illness and complaint imaginable is included with DSM-IV criteria for diagnosis and good guidelines for treatment or referral in each case.

The authors have succeeded in their goal of creating a thorough yet portable guide that should be invaluable to a broad range of practicing clinicians. This text packs a wallop in less than 0.75 MB of memory. As with the other e-books in the HHM series, it also works quite well from an external memory card.

Critical Care Medicine

I would recommend checking the web site for the latest version and other useful and famous titles. My copy of *Critical Care Medicine* (184K, a part of the Current Clinical Strategies series from www.ccspublishing.com) has no bookmarks, and thus, navigation is done by scrolling or using the search feature. This seems a bit cumbersome for such a large document, but you could set your own bookmarks. A lot of information is here and the source, and authors are known, unlike many of the freeware titles.

Little Black Book of Primary Care

This really useful and interesting e-book (4th edition, by Daniel K. Onion, M.D., M.P.H., F.A.C.P., powered by Skyscape) goes beyond the basics. Yes, it has the "usual clinical approaches" for a vast array of medical conditions, and it has a great collection of clinical "pearls." However, it also has more than 6000 specific literature references. This text points you in the right direction to get even more information if you are looking for it. A print version is also available if you want to compare. It goes by the name of "The Complete Guide" and is part of the "Blackwell's Primary Care Essentials" series; however, I don't see how it could beat the handheld version.

An extensive table of contents that is divided into typical medical specialty areas enhances the *Little Black Book*. Moreover, several different indexes exist that expedite navigation: a Main Index, a Prevention Index, and an Emergency Index. More texts should be arranged in such a convenient manner. Maybe we would be able to get to things in a hurry that way.

Ferri's Clinical Advisor: Diseases and Disorders

This is another happy marriage (by Mosby, powered by Skyscape, version 5.0.116/2002.8.22, 2.4MB+ [2400K+], $59.95) between a trusted medical reference and the easy navigability of Skyscape software.

There are several books in the Ferri's series, most of which are available for the PDA through Skyscape. However, I have chosen just one of these as an example.

As with most of the Skyscape medical PDA references, FerriDiseases (as it is listed at the Skyscape web site) is easily navigated by any one of several ways. You can choose to search the Main Index, the ICD-9-CM Index, the Medication Index, or the Table of Contents.

To get an idea of the scope of this reference, let's take a closer look at the table of contents. Interestingly, the table of contents is merely an alphabet with attached "+" signs. For example, tap on the "+" sign next to "D" to reveal an "exploded" view of the applicable table of contents under "D." In this case, 22 different articles (generally each a disease or disorder) from "DeQuervain's tenosynovitis" to "Dystonia" exist.

Besides similar detail for the rest of the alphabet, the table of contents winds up with figures, tables, and boxes. The figures do not show up on my Palm OS device, although the user is given references for most of these. This one small concession was apparently necessary in the transition from print to PDA. However, the other two categories, tables and boxes, contain a wealth of information in a useful, succinct style. There are 111 tables from "Abuse, drug" to "Whiplash injury." Several of the topics require multiple tables. Then there are 67 boxes, including information on subjects from "Abruptio placentae" to "Vaginal bleeding during pregnancy." Spend some time perusing these for a reminder about how much information you have at your fingertips.

Of course, no matter how you navigate FerriDiseases, each disease or disorder entity is further organized in a thorough and logical manner. In each case, Skyscape's patented SmARTbuttons (at the right of the screen) guide you to the relevant points of each article. For example, begin to use Graffiti to write "hep" in the "Look for ______" area of the Main Index. You don't even need to finish the word "hepatitis" before you are taken to that section of the index. You can quickly tap on "Hepatitis C" to go to the article on that subject. SmARTbuttons on the side divide the article up into its applicable components: Definition, Synonyms, ICD-9CM Codes, Basic Information, Diagnosis, Treatment, Pearls/Considerations, References, and (often) the Author. I love this system! I am not forced to scan an entire article to find the information I want now. Instead, I can quickly jump to just the piece of the article that is pertinent to my search. In the case of Hepatitis C, all of the buttons were active because there was information in the article within each button area. In other cases, when no relevant information exists, the specific button indicates this with an "x" so you don't waste your time. Histoplasmosis, for example, has no synonym listed.

As with other Skyscape products, FerriDiseases works just great from external memory card (the .pdb database files). A handy cross-linking feature enables the user to jump quickly to the same subject in another applicable Skyscape product. For example, I was in FerriDiseases/Hepatitis C/Treatment looking at interferon. I tapped the appropriate icon at the top right corner. This gave me a dropdown menu of other Skyscape products that I have installed. I selected DrDrugs (Davis's Drug Guide for Physicians) and was immediately taken to that reference with choices to tap on INH, Ribavirin (or others), and their specific articles in DrDrugs. I can just as easily return to where I left off in FerriDiseases. This is quite a handy feature and recommends highly the convenient use of more than one Skyscape product on the same handheld device.

FerriDiseases is a useful and thorough pocket reference. The depth and breadth of its content has to be seen to be appreciated. The ease of use belies the mass of information you have at your fingertips. Familiarity will make this an indispensable tool.

■ Facts and Comparisons A to Z Drug Facts ("A2zDrugs") and Davis's Drug Guide for Physicians/Facts and Comparisons Drug Interaction Facts ("Dr. Drugs/iFacts")

I apologize in advance for this confusing entry, but the reasons will soon be apparent. Here are two of the many drug references offered by Skyscape and an example of some of the ways you can purchase software bundled together. On the one hand, we see A2zDrugs (version 5.3.126/2002.10.2, powered by Skyscape, 2.9MB+, $49.95) marketed by itself. On the other hand, we see an example of Skyscape bundling two different drug references together even though they are from different publishers (Dr. Drugs/iFacts, version 4.1.33/2001.12.20 and version 4.2.43/2002.1.31, by F.A. Davis and by Facts and Comparisons, respectively, powered by Skyscape, $107 bundled together). This makes perfect sense when one considers how they complement each other. Indeed, Skyscape bundles medical titles together in a multitude of creative and cost-saving ways because they currently have more than 100 medical PDA software titles from which to choose. These are just examples of a couple of the drug reference titles. More in this category and other categories exist, and the reader is directed to the Skyscape web site to sort out the latest selection and prices.

As with any category in which there are multiple titles, I would suggest trying them before you make a purchase decision. This seems particularly appropriate when it comes to drug references. Skyscape makes this easy by offering trial versions of everything available at its web site. Sometimes trial versions are limited versions without all of the entries being active. Sometimes they are limited to a period of time. Either way, this gives you a good chance to see whether a particular title suits your needs better than another.

You may have come to appreciate by now some of the Skyscape features that these titles share with other titles. They also work quite well from an external memory card. This is quite a plus when you want to carry several large references in your PDA. Your internal memory would quickly become the limiting factor. External memory, however, is an expandable resource. You would load up more and/or larger memory cards, just as you might with today's digital cameras.

Furthermore, there's the linking feature between Skyscape products. You could be reading, for example, about hypothyroidism in FerriDiseases. A tap on the linking feature at the top of the page would bring up a menu of other Skyscape products that are accessible on your PDA. If you tapped on either A2zDrugs or Dr. Drugs, you would see a menu of the relevant drugs in the respective database (in this case, Amiodarone, Dopamine, Levothroid, and Levothyroxine). By tapping on the appropriate drug, you could select to read more about Indications, Contraindications and Precautions, Adverse Reactions and Side Effects, Interactions, U.S. Availability, Route and Dosage, U.S. Brand Names, Action, Classification, Pregnancy Risk Factor, Pharmacokinetics, Controlled Substance Schedule, Canadian Brand Names, Lab Test Interferences, and more. Some variation exists in these selections between Dr. Drugs and A2zDrugs, but you would want to check them out individually anyway. It is clear that a lot more information is here at your fingertips than you are likely to get from any of the available free PDA drug references. This is a good reason for a medical professional to choose to pay for one of these drug guides. It is also important to note that you are not bogged down by this information. The SmARTbuttons along the side of the screen allow the user to choose which information to access quickly. You don't have to read an entire treatise on a particular drug to get to the data that you need most urgently. You could then simply tap and link back to your reference in FerriDiseases (e.g., if that's where you started and you wanted to get back to your reading on hypothyroidism).

The beauty of these various products is how well they integrate with each other and how the user can jump between them. This is a real plus for the entire product line. It is especially elegant in its execution when we consider the third piece of the software that I include in this listing. Remember the previously mentioned bundle of Dr. Drugs/iFacts? If you had installed these products to your PDA, you could jump from FerriDiseases to Dr. Drugs, find your appropriate drug, and also link to iFacts, which, in turn, allows the user to access rapidly any drug/drug interactions that might apply to any given patient situation. Merely check the appropriate boxes of all of the medications being used by your patient, or skip to a drop down menu of all of the drugs that interact with Levothyroxine, for example. Using this kind of information from this kind of database surely will soon become the standard of care. I doubt that tomorrow's juries will have much sympathy for clinicians who do not use this type of program. What better way to access this data than through your PDA?

Taber's Cyclopedic Medical Dictionary

Although I have been a big fan of *Taber's* (edition 19, 2001, by F.A. Davis Co. [5300K or 5.3MB]) for years in the print version, you can now have this authoritative reference in your PDA. It is easily searched and handy and has thorough entries. Figure 115 shows the table of contents, a sample page, and the navigation tools for this text reader.

Similar to several of the products mentioned here, *Taber's* uses the HandHeldMed Reader. Once you know how to navigate one text in this format, you know how to get around in all of them. This is a really useful reference to have, as long as you have sufficient memory to do the job. Large texts require lots of memory. My advice is to store texts such as this in external (add-on) memory, as they work just

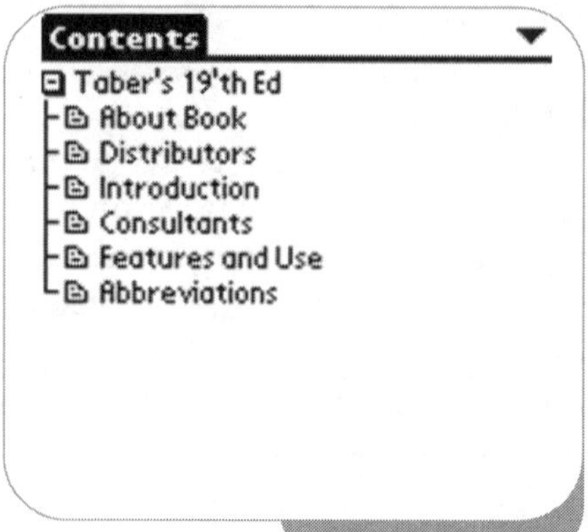
Contents
Taber's 19'th Ed
About Book
Distributors
Introduction
Consultants
Features and Use
Abbreviations

Figure 115A

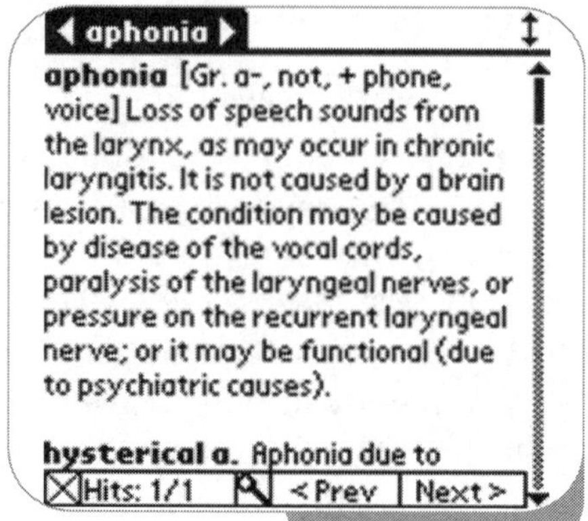
aphonia
aphonia [Gr. a-, not, + phone, voice] Loss of speech sounds from the larynx, as may occur in chronic laryngitis. It is not caused by a brain lesion. The condition may be caused by disease of the vocal cords, paralysis of the laryngeal nerves, or pressure on the recurrent laryngeal nerve; or it may be functional (due to psychiatric causes).
hysterical a. Aphonia due to
Hits: 1/1
<Prev
Next>

Figure 115B

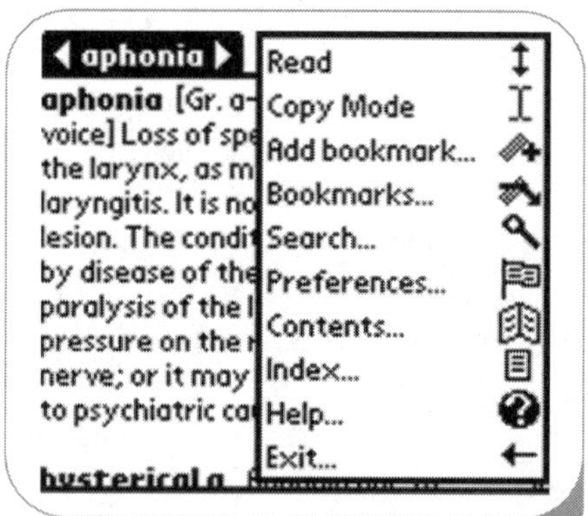
aphonia
Read
Copy Mode
Add bookmark...
Bookmarks...
Search...
Preferences...
Contents...
Index...
Help...
Exit...

Figure 115C

fine from there, thus preserving your internal PDA memory for other things that do not work from external memory.

Stedman's Concise Medical Dictionary

Don't let the word "concise" in the title of this product fool you. This electronic marvel for the PDA is likely to be the only medical dictionary that you will ever need. The print version of *Stedman's* (4th edition, Lippincott Williams & Wilkins, powered by Skyscape, $39.95) has been a well-trusted medical reference for a long time. The concise version seems a successful attempt to make the old standby more user friendly. This electronic version accomplishes something that even the concise print version could not: It is quite portable.

As with other Skyscape medical PDA products, the controls are instantly familiar. All of the usual conveniences of the format and search engine are consistent from product to product throughout the Skyscape line (now totaling more than 100 medical titles). Patented SmARTbuttons on the side of the screen guide the user quickly to different views. Dropdown information boxes explain the various SmARTbuttons if you ever forget their functions. Searching is quick and easy by simply using Graffiti or the keyboard to insert your desired word. The search begins before you even complete the word, often making it unnecessary to complete the input. Definitions are thorough and informative, just what we have come to expect from *Stedman's*.

Weighing in at a whopping 7800K of memory (nearly 8MB), it is a good thing that *Stedman's* works so well from external memory. In fact, this is where I store all of my Skyscape products.

Here is a tip for installing these large e-book files to the handheld: I found that I was often without sufficient internal memory to make such an installation to my PDA. I now use a separate USB external memory card reader (my model reads six varieties, including Compact Flash, Secure Digital, Multi-Media Cards, and Memory Sticks). The card reader is attached directly to my PC via a USB connector, acts just like another drive, and requires no software or installation. I install the kind of memory card that my PDA can use (currently a Memory Stick for my Sony Clie NX-60) in the reader and install the e-book directly from the PC to the memory card, bypassing the PDA altogether. This works quite nicely for large files and frees me from the worry of how much internal memory I have left on my PDA.

Dorland's Pocket Medical Dictionary

This offering completes the trio of commonly cited medical dictionaries. Which one you choose to carry with you is really a matter of individual taste. *Dorland's* (by W.B. Saunders, powered by Skyscape, version 4.0.33/2001.12.20), like *Stedman's* and *Taber's*, has earned its share of the market over the years. I like them all and find them quite comparable to the print versions, yet infinitely more portable, searchable, and useful.

Dorland's is simply organized around the "Look for ____" feature. You search the Main Index in this fashion, just as you would look something up in a print dictionary. Here you have the added advantage that the PDA version will electronically finish the word for you, thereby greatly speeding up your searches. As with other Skyscape products, a further advantage is that *Dorland's* can be accessed easily while in another Skyscape product. Conversely, you can "link out" from a *Dorland's* word search to the relevant entry in another Skyscape product that you have installed on your PDA.

Dorland's is, as you would expect from a medical dictionary, a large text. However, only the 161K operating program needs to be installed in your handheld's internal memory. The 5.4 MB database works quite comfortably from an external memory card.

DeGowin and DeGowin's Diagnostic Examination

This text fills a unique niche in medical PDA e-books, concerning itself mainly with the diagnostic examination of the patient. The fact that it is based on the 1994 print edition (6th edition, 1994, by McGraw-Hill/Handheldmed [695K]) should be of little concern because exam techniques and the thought processes behind them are largely unchanged. More important, I think, is the fact that this is the 6th edition of a reliable text that has earned a respected reputation since 1965. In those days, it was known as *DeGowin's Bedside Diagnostic Examination.*

DeGowin's is organized into an introduction, 12 chapters, and a bibliography. It proceeds in a logical manner to guide the user through a well-organized, head-to-toe examination and review of laboratory studies. Included are core techniques of eliciting the medical history, methods of physical examination, relevant anatomy, and a stepwise approach. This is a text for both student and seasoned professional clinicians. It is both a learning tool and a reminder of the way things should be done. Even as an experienced professional, one may be called on to perform a rarely used test or technique. How do we remember them? I find myself relying on just such PDA texts as *DeGowin's*.

As with the other HHM texts, *DeGowin's* works well from an external memory card. The search feature is a handy way to find a specific topic, test, technique, or body part. I still like to browse the table of contents, which is organized and logical in its arrangement. As a clinical instructor, *DeGowin's* is close to my heart, and as a clinician, I find that it serves a very useful function as well.

Beiks Products

BDicty is the crown jewel of the Beiks line of handheld software (www.beiks.com). It is probably the leading dictionary application for PDAs. Beiks has taken one simple concept and gotten it right. Their BDicty has become a platform capable of carrying a myriad of "lexicons." This way, you can have BDicty installed on your device and select from any number of references that you have installed to it. For example, you might want to refer to a Spanish–English lexicon to help your communications with a Hispanic patient. Similarly, within BDicty, you can jump to a medical dictionary, a medical encyclopedia, or a medical abbreviations dictionary.

I found the navigation a little less intuitive than it might have been, but the Beiks Company provides a good instruction manual that answers all of my questions. The medical products mentioned previously may be geared more to the lay user than the medical professional but have several important features. For one, they pack a surprising number of entries into a small amount of memory. These programs also accomplish their task at a relatively inexpensive price. I think this is somewhat because of the modular nature of the products. Lexicons appear to be generally well written, and the system is ultimately user friendly.

If you don't have a lot of room to spare in your PDA but still want a handy medical dictionary, I think the Beiks BDicty with the medical dictionary installed is a worthy addition. For a little more memory, you could opt for the medical encyclopedia installation instead. It seems to have the content of the medical dictionary plus more. I also like the medical abbreviations dictionary just because it seems like I'm forever seeking clarification of some abbreviation.

Best of all, if you want to conserve precious internal memory on your PDA, you will be happy to know that the Beiks lexicons work fine from external memory (SD, Memory Stick, etc.) as long as the platform BDicty is maintained on the internal memory. This means that you can have the very small BDicty (59K) in your main memory and several texts (medical dictionary, 2.8MB; medical encyclopedia, 3.5MB; medical abbreviations dictionary, 650K, one or more foreign language dictionaries, etc.) stored in your add-on memory.

Beiks also has other products that are worth exploring and trying on their web page. They have a host of foreign language lexicons for BDicty. Besides helping with your patient encounters, these might be useful considerations for foreign travel. They also produce a very interesting program, called Woman, which combines desktop features with PDA portability features. With Woman, the user tracks multiple features of her menstrual cycle to help conveniently predict fertility for conception, to avoid conception, or even to plan for better vacations. It is beautifully done with color graphics and multiple calendars that synchronize between desktop and handheld smoothly. I think that this would be a fine product to recommend to female patients or couples. It's a great way to empower patients to be more involved in their own health care.

In addition, new from Beiks, I've been trying out a new class of products: talking phrasebooks. I am fascinated by the potential of this newest piece of technology. With Beiks Talking Spanish Phrasebook, I am able to select an English phrase and tap on it, and then my PDA will translate the phrase and audibly speak it. To be sure, you must have one of the newest PDAs in order to take advantage of this feature (like the Sony Clie PEG-NX60 or NX70 or the Palm Tungsten). Nevertheless, if you really want to impress your colleagues, simply tap your PDA to have it speak in Spanish. Of course, Beiks has other languages available too. As with their other lexicons, the large files required of speaking phrasebooks are easily accommodated in external memory. I can see significant applicability with these products and patients to whom English is a second or foreign language. These talking phrase books could really help to bridge a gap.

STATCoder Series

These products are powered by TealInfo and are all quite useful and unique (three separate products: STAT E&M Coder, STAT ICD-9 Coder, STAT CPT Coder, available from http://www.statcoder.com). They seem to fill a void in the billing and coding area. Here are a few screen shots of STAT E&M Coder in action. First, you see the menu to select what type of patient visit this is (Figure 116). If you were to select Office New, you would then begin to do the H&P and tap on history questions asked and exam elements performed.

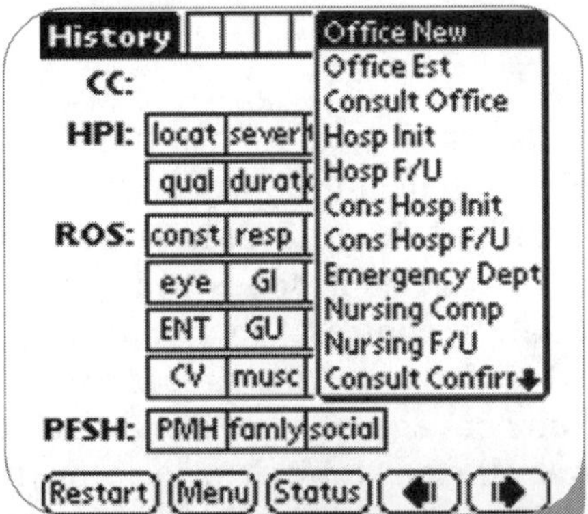

Figure 116A

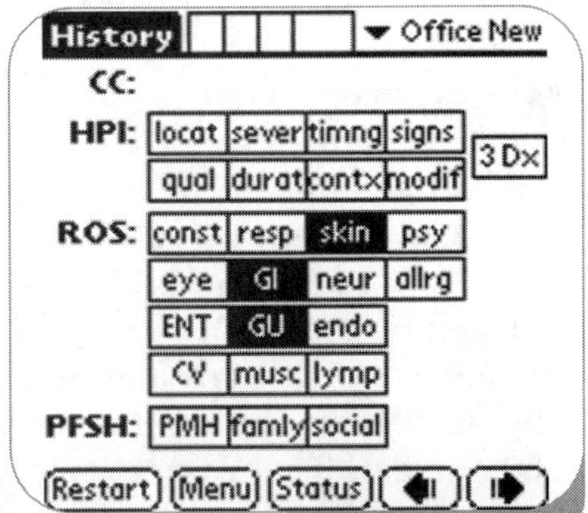

Figure 116B

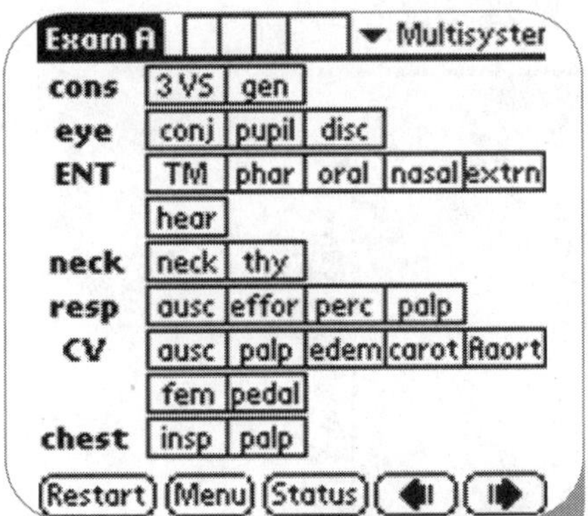

Figure 116C

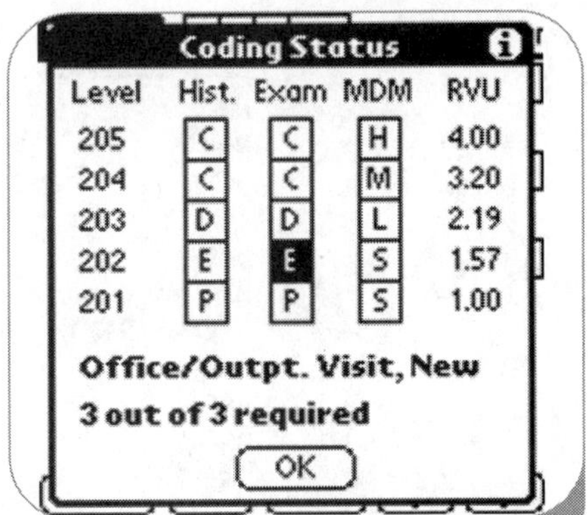

Figure 116D

At any point, you could tap on Status, and the Coding Status would pop up to give you a summary of where you are and/or what elements you would still need to do to improve your coding level. You can see how this program could easily pay for itself in a very short while.

The site (www.statcoder.com) also features several free PDA tools of interest: STAT Cholesterol, STAT GrowthCharts, STAT Cardiac Clearance, and GRACE ACS Risk. These free offerings all are specialized medical calculators. The latter is a predictor of in-hospital mortality (acute coronary syndrome) in the Global Registry of Acute Coronary Events risk model. The STAT folks have even been kind enough to bundle all of their free programs into one convenient package for downloading called the "Clinical Productivity Set."

MobileEMS

This is one of my favorite commercial medical products, and it also comes at a great price for what you get. Mobile EMS (formerly PalmEMS, version 3.0, 2001, www.emszone.com, Jones and Bartlett Publishers, Inc., 1322 records, $24.95), in contrast to what its name implies, is a program for any medical professional. It claims over 1300 entries. It is easily navigable by seven convenient tabs along the side of the screen. They respectively display the master index, an acronym index, an algorithm index, an anatomical diagrams index, a calculator index, a prescription index, and a treatment index (Figure 117).

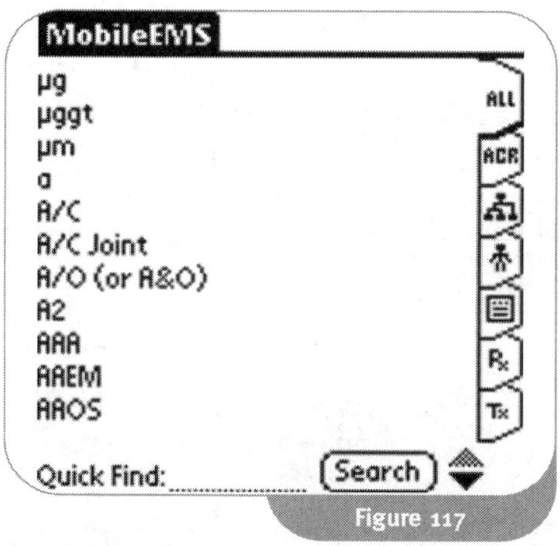

Figure 117

Each of these tabs reveals a large number of entries in each of the indexes. Especially unique are the algorithms, the calculators, and the anatomical diagrams (Figure 118).

My favorites are the anatomical diagrams. Besides being good memory aids, these can be useful for explaining things to patients. The drawings are very nicely done and not extremely detailed but are useful in their simplicity. An anatomy "tap map" lets you zero in on spe-

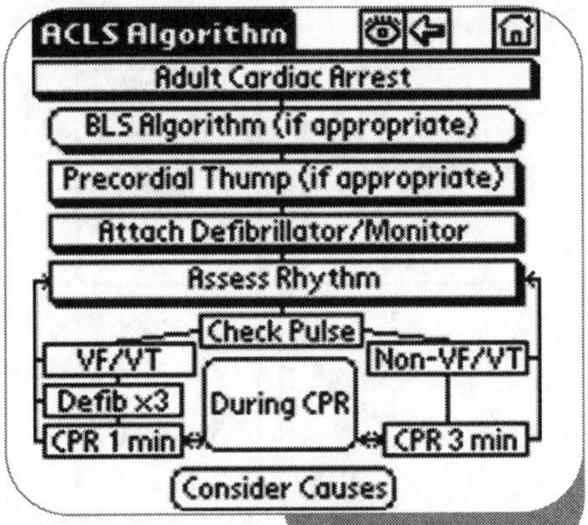

Figure 118A

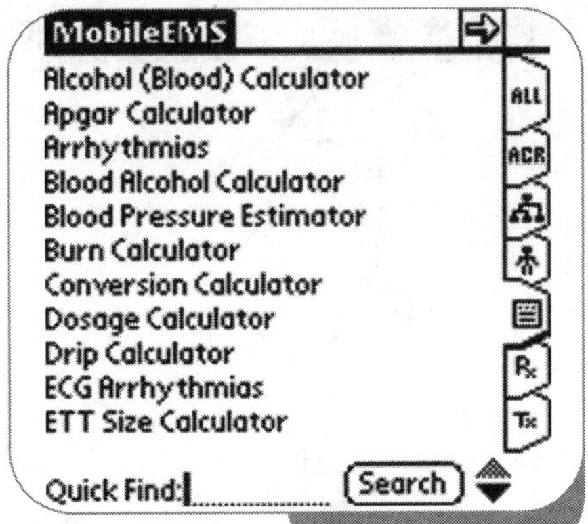

Figure 118B

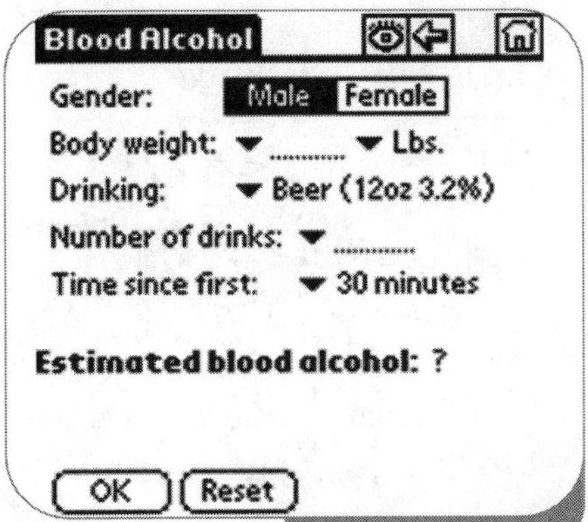

Figure 118C

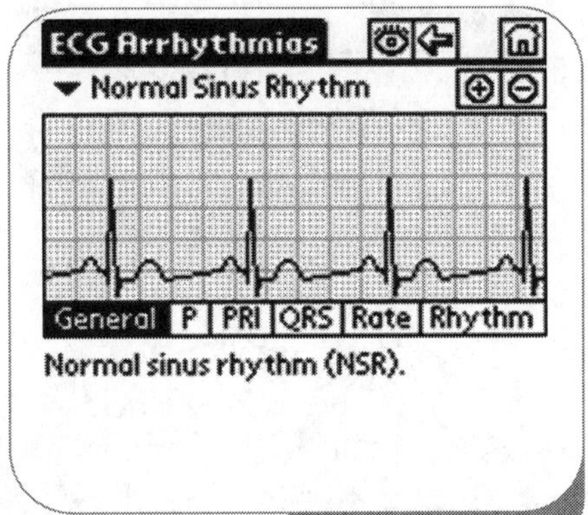

Figure 118D

cific areas of the anatomy. Some of the drawings also feature a zoom out feature for extra views. MobileEMS also includes an anatomy chart of those pesky anatomical directions (e.g., proximal, distal, medial, and lateral). This can be especially useful for students of medicine (Figure 119).

Additionally, the program features other navigational aids that help to speed things up. A Quick Find (search) function helps to avoid so much scrolling. If an item has related material in another article, you can jump to the related material quickly with a small "eye" icon in the upper right-hand corner of the screen. Finally, there is another search feature that allows you to search the entire database or any individual tab category of the database. This is very well thought out.

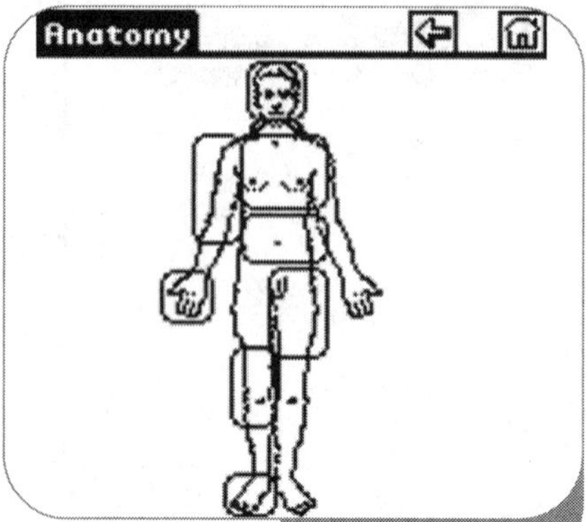

Figure 119A

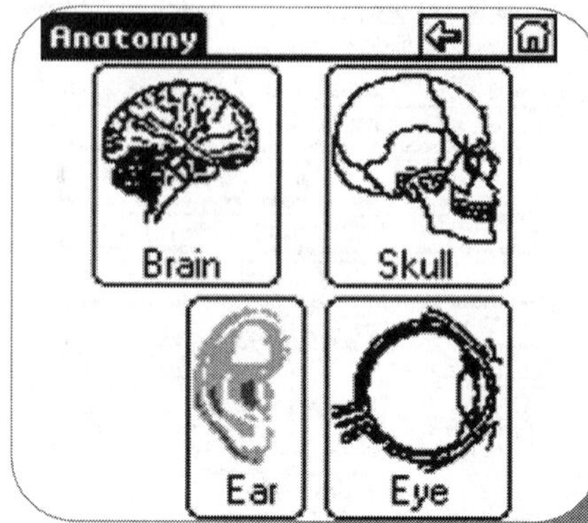

Figure 119B

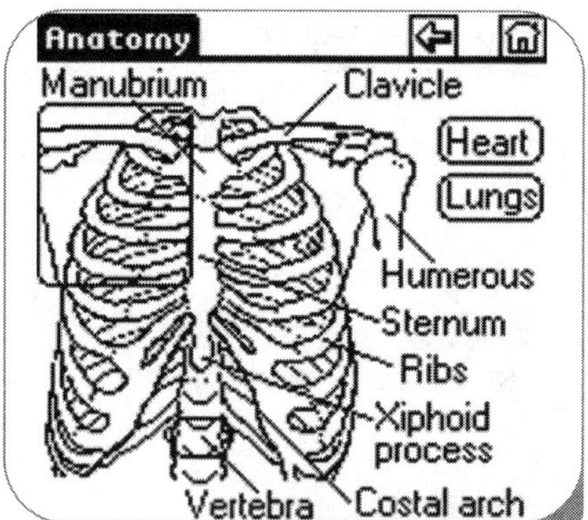

Figure 119C

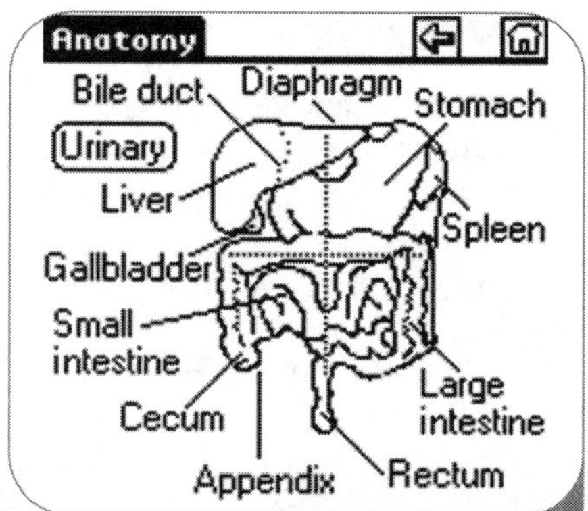

Figure 119D

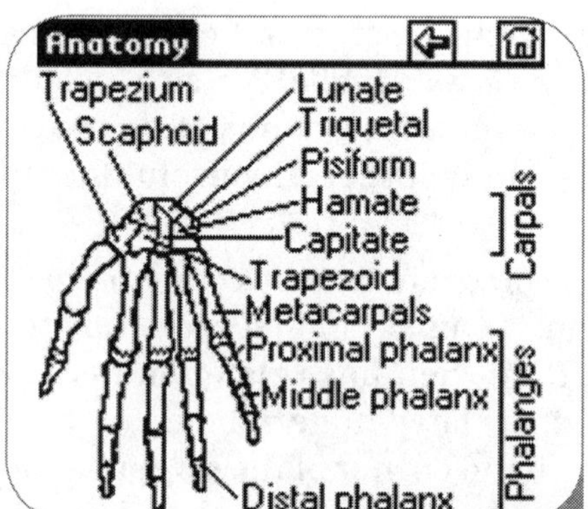

Figure 119E

RN-Emerg

I have the trial version of this program, which I like very much. I can't imagine how the full commercial version could pack more information. RN-Emerg (version 1.02, 2002, by Palmtree.ca ltd, available at www.palmgear.com or www.handango.com) is another program whose name belies its content and its usefulness. I feel that this program has broad applicability to a wide range of medical professionals and students.

RN-Emerg features eight big, graphic, handy tabs. One each exists for ECG strips, Calculations, MI/ST elevation, a calculator for common Med drips, an ACLS quick ref, a Peds/OBS calculator, a tracker for your Continuing ed, and a Shift log. I say the tabs are big and handy because they are actually large enough to tap with your fingertip (cringe) if necessary (Figure 120).

Fifteen different ECG strips with graphics, criteria, five commonly used calculations, and 17 common med drip calculators are available. The ACLS quick reference seems quite handy and useful (although no source reference is available). The Peds/OBS tab features seven handy calculators of its own: APGAR, pregnancy wheel, neonate resuscitation guidelines, pediatric rule of nines (for burns), peds danger signs, peds weight calculator/vital signs, and an acetaminophen/ibuprofen calculator. This is all very handy. RN-Emerg has a lot of useful information that is easily accessible and all in one place.

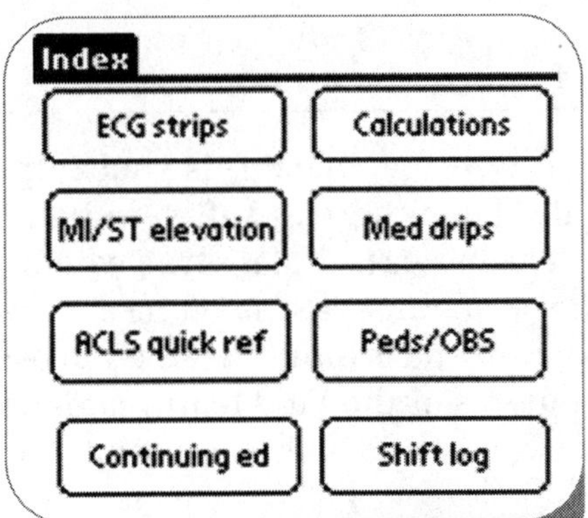

Figure 120A

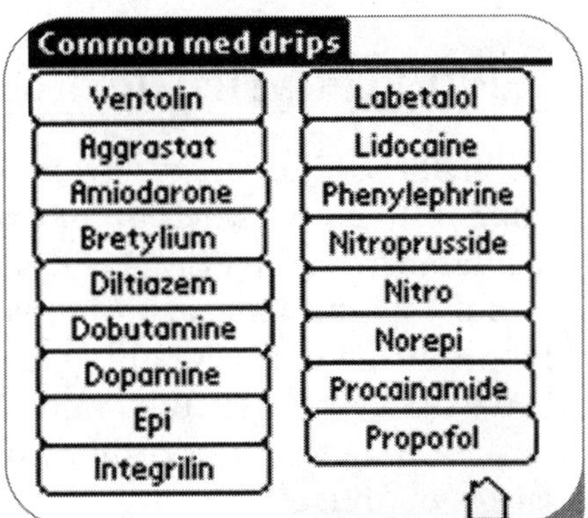

Figure 120B

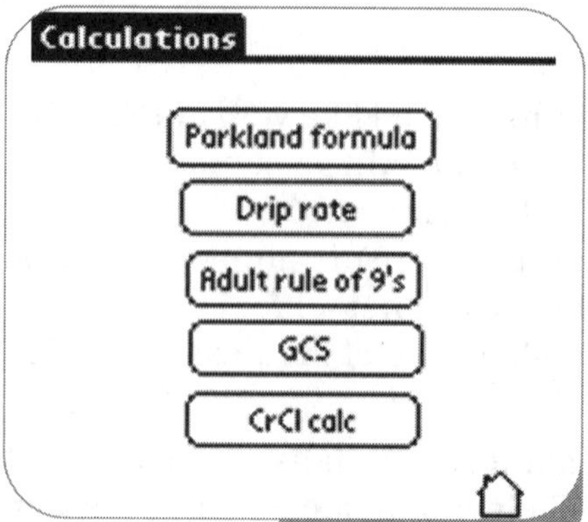

Figure 120C

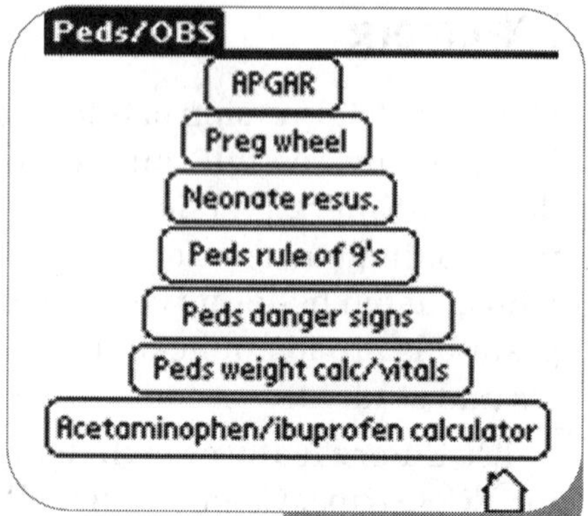

Figure 120D

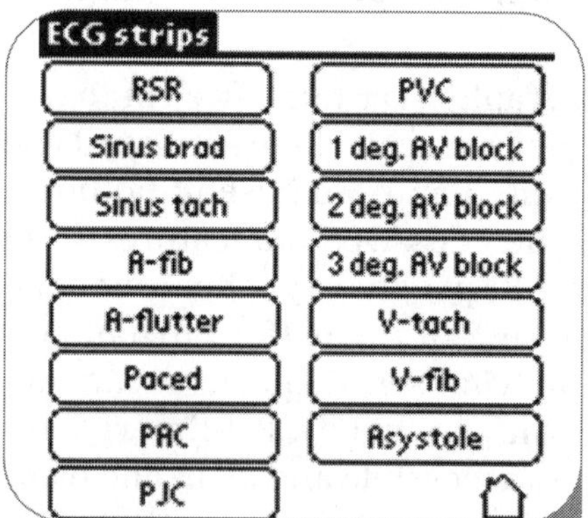

Figure 120E

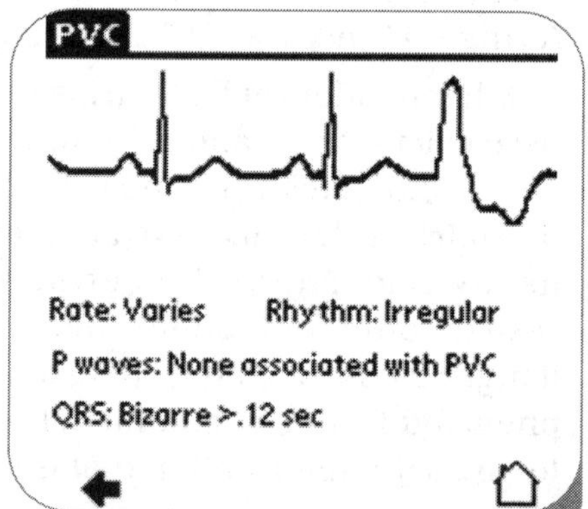

Figure 120F

PEPID/PEPID Free Toxicology

PEPID Free Toxicology (available at www.pepid.com) is your introduction to an entire suite of excellent commercial software that is available from the PEPID web site. The bonus is that it's free whether or not you purchase any of the other programs. As you can see from Figure 121, it is a very complete program and is intuitively easy to use. You can navigate via the table of contents or the Find feature. Figure 121 shows a small portion of what you would see if you tapped on Drugs of Abuse.

Figure 122 shows a portion of what you would see if you pursued Ethanol in that category. The entries that follow are short, succinct

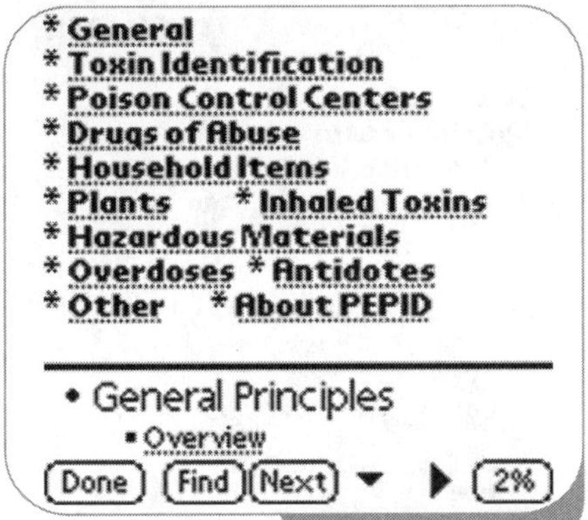

Figure 121A

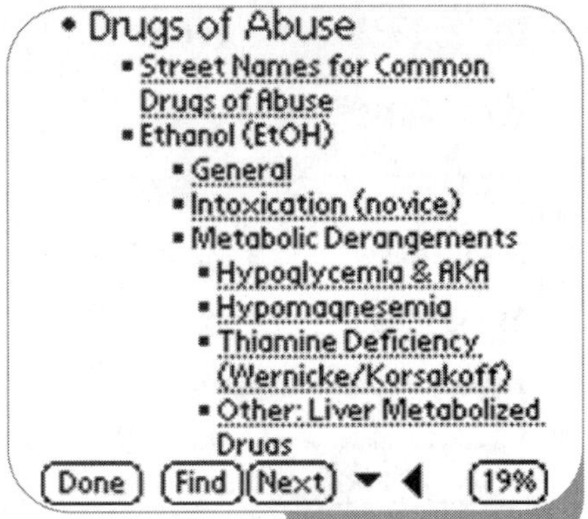
• Drugs of Abuse
▪ Street Names for Common Drugs of Abuse
▪ Ethanol (EtOH)
▪ General
▪ Intoxication (novice)
▪ Metabolic Derangements
▪ Hypoglycemia & AKA
▪ Hypomagnesemia
▪ Thiamine Deficiency (Wernicke/Korsakoff)
▪ Other: Liver Metabolized Drugs
Done Find Next 19%
Figure 121B

bullets in outline form. They are easy to access, important, and full of need-to-know information. This is both a great introduction to other PEPID programs and a great stand-alone program.

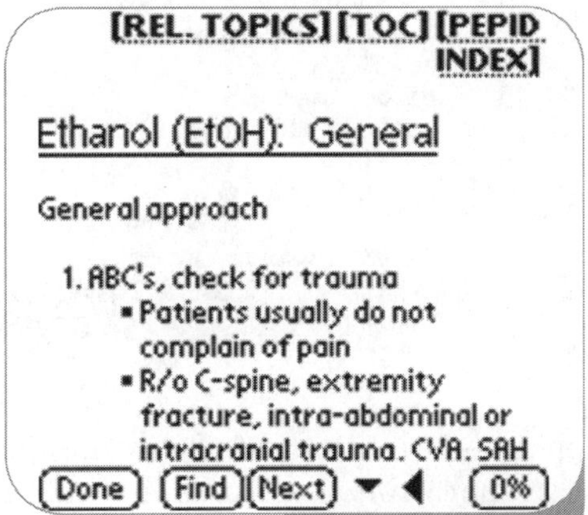

Figure 122

The PEPID site also includes several fine commercial offerings to consider, depending on what type of medical professional you are. Figure 123 illustrates some of the content of the PEPID ED version.

QuizApp

Although not strictly a medical software application, QuizApp (version 2.0.4 by AdroitMobile) has sufficient medical modules available that it should be included in this section of the book. As its name

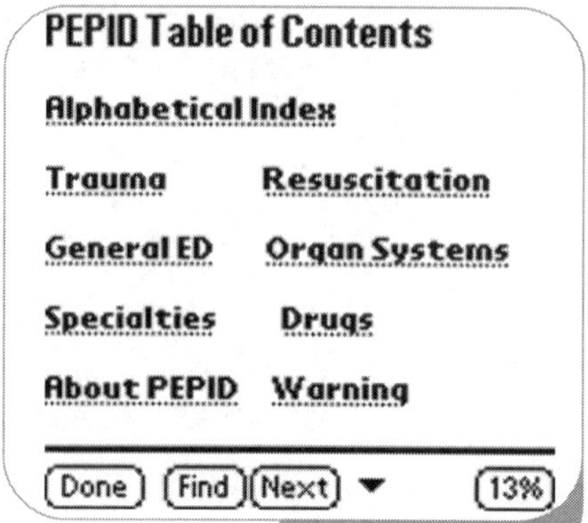

Figure 123A

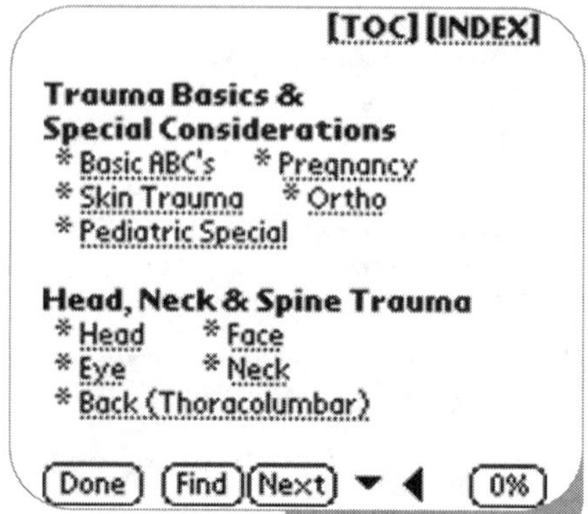

Figure 123B

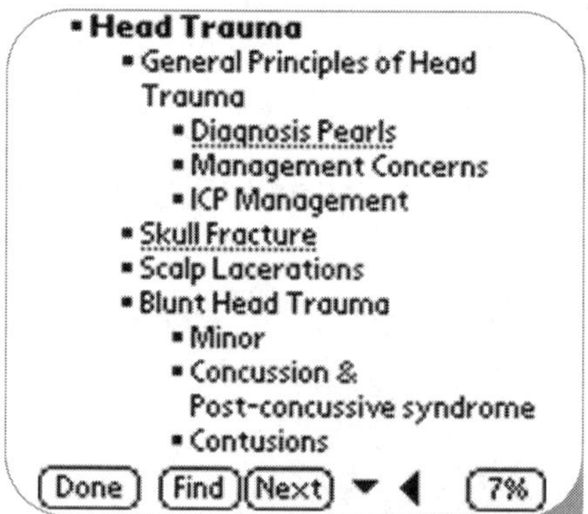

Figure 123C

implies, QuizApp is self-quizzing software. The makers call it "Test Prep To Go," and it performs that function quite nicely. You download the free QuizApp and then add various free or commercial "modules" for quizzing yourself in a variety of areas. For example, a free American Sign Language module or free Basic Spanish Verb Flashcards are available (Figure 124).

Among the more medically oriented modules is an entire series called Games4Doctors, which includes such modules as Anatomy, Physiology, Internal Medicine, Emergency Medicine, Pediatrics, History of Medicine, and others. Quizzes are set up as sessions, and the software keeps track of your score and areas of strength and weakness. This is great preparation for board exams. You can easily have

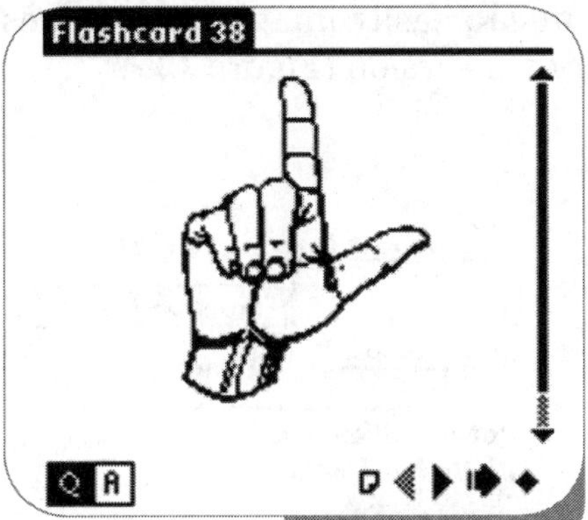

Figure 124A

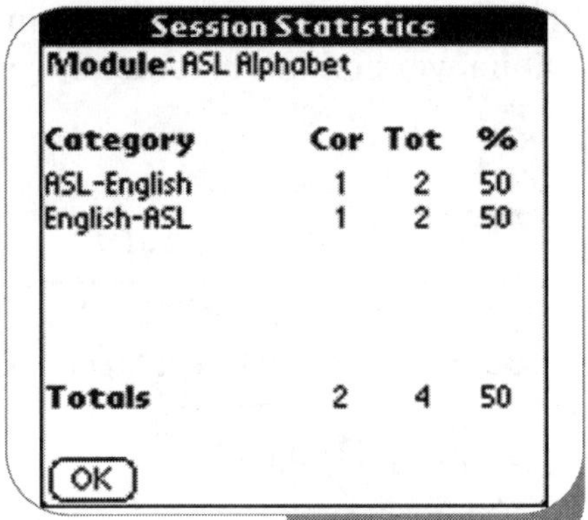

Figure 124B

a quiz session while waiting for a plane or challenge a colleague to a game of medical trivia. QuizApp is a fun learning tool that I recommend to my students.

Patient Tracking Databases: HandEchart and Others

Patient Tracking represents an entire category of medical PDA software. As the name of the category suggests, it allows you to do a multitude of patient-tracking functions. Some of the titles to look for are Patient Tracker, Patient Keeper, and Ward Watch. Here I review HandEchart because I helped to author this software. This is the patient-tracking software that our physician assistant students have been field testing for the past few years. I am unabashedly proud of it and know it better than any of the other available software in this category.

HandEchart is available from www.ddhsoftware.com, the folks who brought you HanDbase (previously reviewed). We developed it for our physician assistant students to record and track their clinical patient encounters. With very simple taps of the stylus, a student is able to record his or her patient encounter in just 1 to 3 minutes. The clinician records patient demographics (age, race, and gender) and then such details as Primary Diagnosis (from a linked ICD-9 Code database) and any procedures performed (from another linked database). The linked database features easily allow the user to tap on choices that can be referenced by a simple lookup feature. The version shown here is the student version, but you can easily imagine the professional version or customizing your own version (Figure 125).

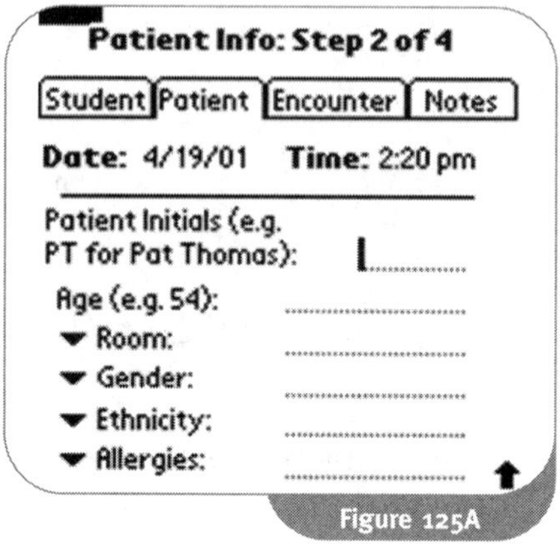

Figure 125A

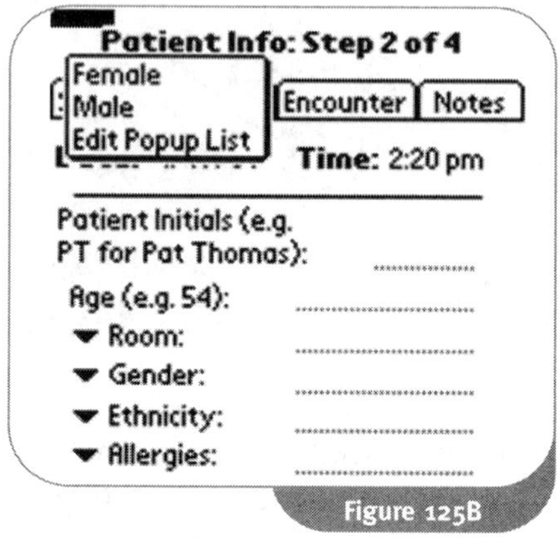

Figure 125B

In Figure 125A you can see the four access tabs across the top of the screen. Here we are in tab 2, having already entered the student information. Now we begin to enter the patient demographics. In Figure 124B, you can see one of the dropdown menus that make the data entry so much faster. These occur wherever you see the small arrows to the left of an entry (Figure 126).

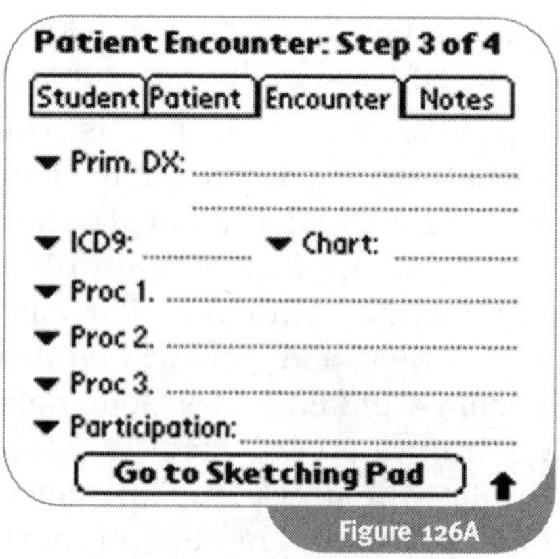

Figure 126A

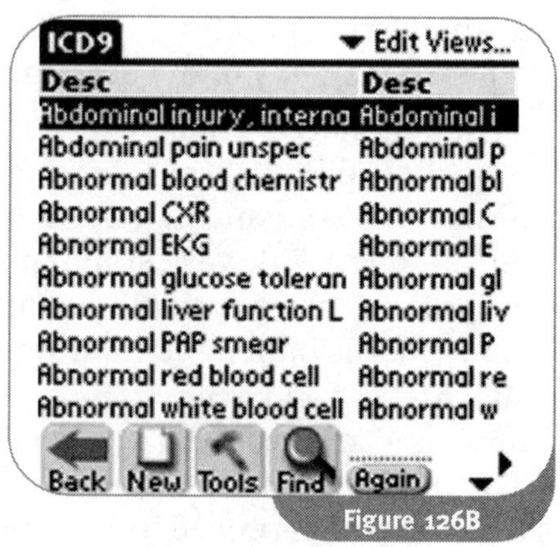

Figure 126B

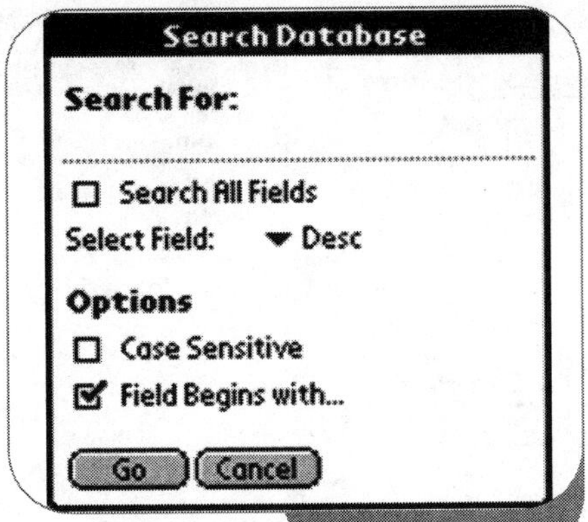

Figure 126C

Figure 126A shows the third access tab, the patient Encounter tab. If you tap on the Primary Diagnosis area, you will come to the linked ICD-9 code database shown in Figure 126B. You can see a faster way to search the ICD-9 code database in Figure 126C.

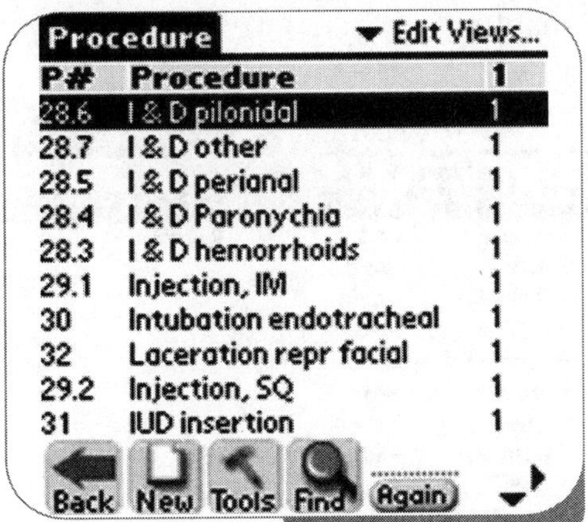

Figure 127

Similarly, the clinician indicates Procedures performed by tapping on that area (as seen in Figure 127) and chooses from the associated linked database of procedures shown in Figure 127. Finally, the user has the option of going to the fourth tab, the Notes (Figure 128). Several choices exist on this page.

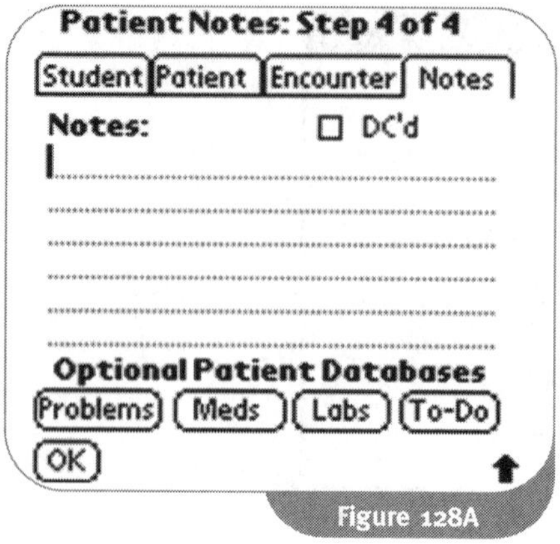

Figure 128A

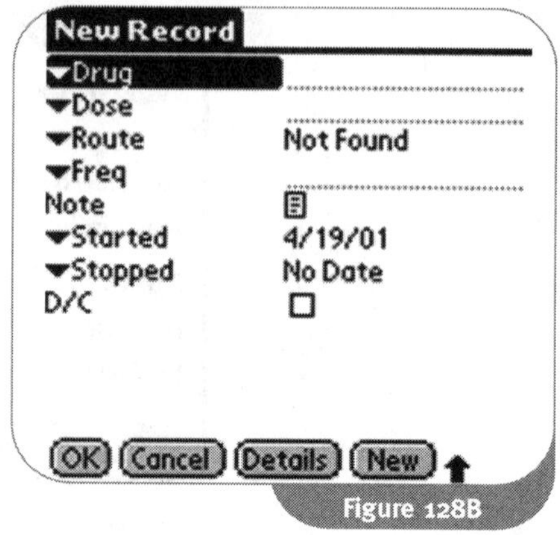

Figure 128B

The user might want to indicate the medications that the patient is on by selecting the Meds button (Figure 128A). This would bring up the page shown in Figure 128B. A tap on the Drug arrow shown there will bring the user to a brief linked DrugList database (shown in Figure 129A). This is just for convenience and is completely customizable by the user. Figure 129B shows a similar process directed to labs and laboratory results.

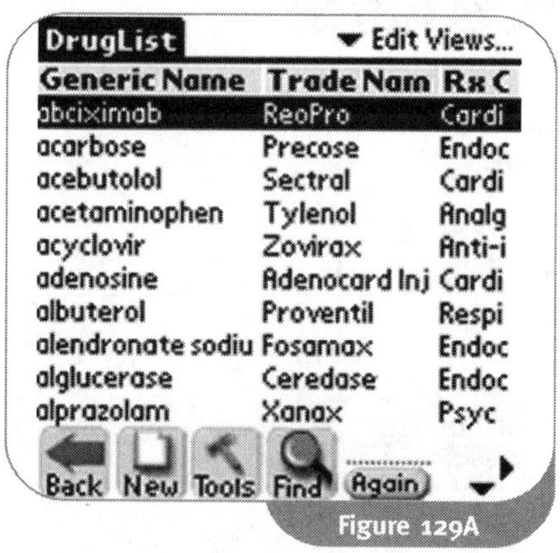

Figure 129A

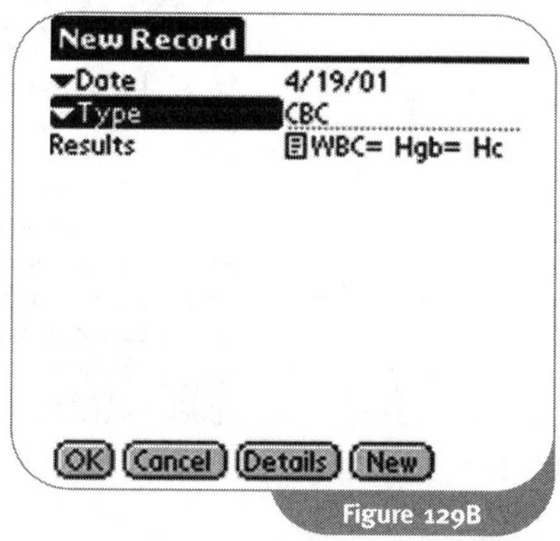

Figure 129B

The point of all of this is to show how a patient tracking database can easily take the place of all of those handwritten note cards and illegible scraps of paper. This makes patient data much more accessible and searchable. You can even print lists or beam the data to a colleague who is taking over your service. There is also great capability to generate reports, which is an added bonus for our physician assistant students. We can even merge data from an entire class of students to generate group statistics. When it comes to future needs for job search purposes or hospital credentialing, the kind of data that this kind of patient tracking can produce from the PDA is invaluable.

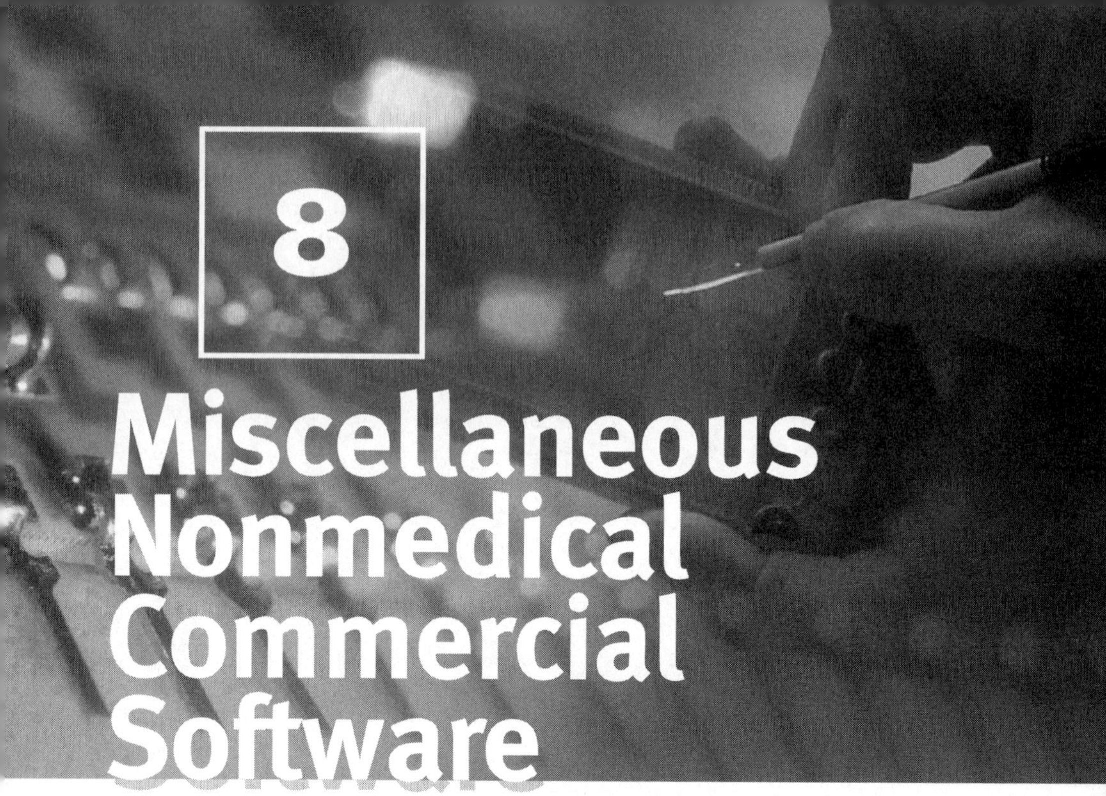

8 Miscellaneous Nonmedical Commercial Software

Some things are useful enough that they are worth paying for them. Moreover, useful software doesn't even have to be medically oriented. Maybe it's simply a program that just makes your job easier or your life simpler. These are some of the programs that I have found to belong in that category. Maybe you can live without them, but I know I'd have a harder time without them. Therefore, I share them with you here.

UnDupe by Stevens Creek Software

My version is an old one (version 1.6) that takes up only 12K of memory. This program does one thing and does it well. It removes duplicate entries from your PDA's Date Book, Address Book, Memo Pad, To Do List, or all four of them at one time. Now, if this is not a problem for you, then congratulations because you don't need this software. After years of HotSyncing with my own and shared departmental Outlook calendars and contact lists, duplicate entries became a huge problem for me. Luckily, a program was available that would clean up the mess. UnDupe scans any or all of the files listed previously here. You can elect for it to just search for the duplicates or find and remove them. I now do this periodically and keep my address book and calendar much cleaner.

Documents To Go

If you do any writing on your PC in Microsoft Word or Microsoft Works or create any spreadsheets using Microsoft Excel, then this program is for you. Documents To Go (by DataViz, www.dataviz.com) takes any of the files that you designate and instantly converts them to PDA-readable files for download to your handheld. More than that, if you make changes to the originals on your PC or on your PDA, the next HotSync will automatically implement the edits for you. You can choose to have the handheld overwrite the desktop, the desktop overwrite the handheld, or synchronize them both. This has proved such an invaluable program that the software is increasingly being bundled with new PDAs. The composition of many documents, especially spreadsheets, is especially tedious on a PDA. Now you don't have to do that. You can compose items on your PC and simply use Documents To Go to make the conversion.

Also, Documents To Go even has a mechanism so that you can share your converted documents with other PDA users even if they don't have Documents To Go. If you have a registered version of Documents To Go, you can beam a colleague the reader called Word To Go first and then beam them the document. Your colleague will be able to, in turn, view the document but will not be able to change it or beam it to another user. For that, they would have to buy their own copy of Documents To Go. This is exceptional on-the-go technology that has saved me a lot of work. A version now comes bundled free with the newer Sony Clie NX models and the Palm Tungsten.

Word Complete

I love this program, although I know others who simply find it annoying. It all depends on your style. Word Complete (by Communication Intelligence Corporation, available at www.shopcic.com, $24.99), once installed and activated on your handheld, helps you to enter text faster. Whether you use Graffiti, a popup keyboard, or an add-on keyboard, this program anticipates the word you have begun to enter, then displays a popup box of possible words for you to choose in lieu of continuing to peck out the rest of the word. Let me show you. First, install the program, and then open it. Check the "Enable" box, and set your rules for its use, as shown in Figure 130.

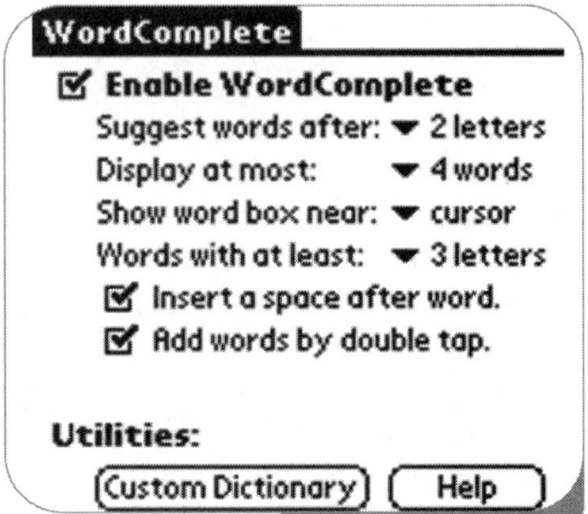
WordComplete
Enable WordComplete
Suggest words after: 2 letters
Display at most: 4 words
Show word box near: cursor
Words with at least: 3 letters
Insert a space after word.
Add words by double tap.
Utilities:
Custom Dictionary
Help
Figure 130

For example, let's say you were going to begin a new memo called "Birthday List." As you begin to enter the word "Birthday," you would start with "Bi" and, because those were the rules we chose in the setup, Word Complete would display a popup of possible choices to complete the word (Figure 131).

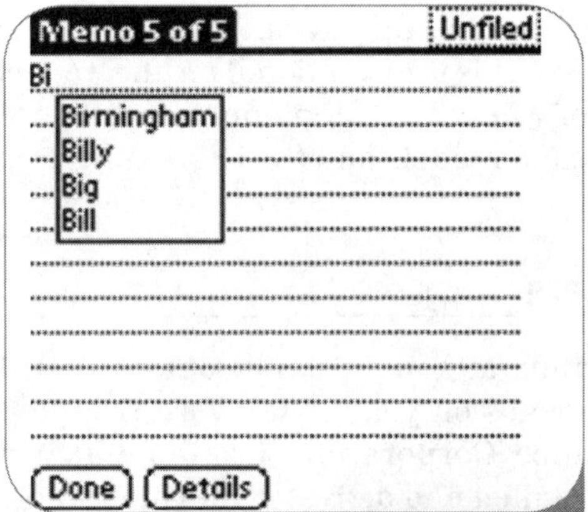

Figure 131

If none of the four choices displayed are the "Birthday" that you were intending to write, keep writing and add an "r." Then you see a new popup as Word Complete zeroes in on the word you really wanted. Now you see it (Figure 132).

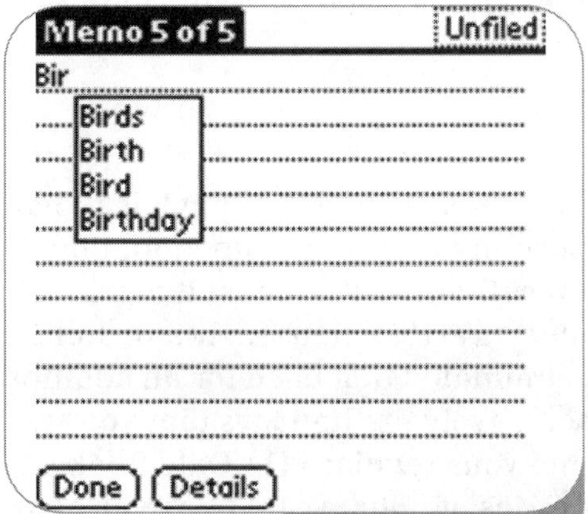

Figure 132

If you tap on the word "Birthday" in the popup list, you have saved yourself five letters of Graffiti input. This can add up, repeatedly, to faster input. You can even add your own customized dictionary of frequently used words. You can choose to have the popup box appear in a different place or you can enable or disable the program as you choose. To me, it is truly amazing how this program seems to anticipate my words so often and how I use it almost without noticing it.

Palm Print/Print Boy

These are two different products. I just mention them both here because they perform the same function. Others may be available by now, too. I think they are nothing short of amazing. I'm most familiar with PalmPrint by Stevens Creek Software. Again, as with other offerings by them that I have written about, they do one thing and do it well. Did you know that you could print output directly from your PDA to a printer, without a computer and without any connecting cables? Well, you can, and it is a real showstopper, not to mention pretty handy. The key is one of the previously named programs, the infrared beaming window on your PDA, and an infrared equipped printer. I have used mine to print directly from the PDA's Memo Pad to a small portable printer (with infrared port) that was originally designed to be used with a laptop computer. You can set margins and choose from several fonts and sizes and between portrait and landscape page orientation and more. This is a very versatile tool.

HoliDates

This is a small, inexpensive program that has proved to be quite useful. I constantly use my Date Book function; however, I was always bothered by the fact that I had to consult a print format calendar in order to determine exactly when the major holidays would occur. Well, HoliDates eliminated that need for an additional calendar. You use it to insert selectively the holidays that you want (or you can do them all) right into your regular PDA Date Book. How handy is that? You can delete entries of holidays that have already occurred, select major religious holidays to insert, and more. Again, this is a versatile and handy program.

Salary Utility

This small, free program (version 2.1, approximately 37K of memory, by Witkowski-Design, this program and other software titles available at www.handgems.com/calculator.html) is actually a calculator. It can compare the various elements of up to five different job offers to help you determine whether that new job offer at a $25,000 increase is really a promotion. This is an especially useful program for new graduates or anybody who is contemplating a move and needs an objective look at the salary facts. You just plug in the components, and the calculator comes up with an hourly rate for comparison (Figure 133).

Word Smith

If you envision your PDA performing more like a real word processor, in the manner that your PC does, then this is the program for you. You can make Word Smith (version 2.1.6, 2002, by Blue Nomad and Quick Sense Software) the default setting for your PDA Memo

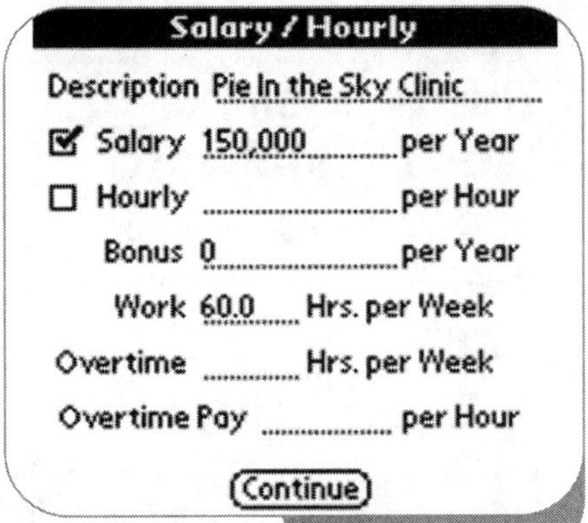
Salary / Hourly
Description Pie In the Sky Clinic
Salary 150,000 per Year
Hourly per Hour
Bonus 0 per Year
Work 60.0 Hrs. per Week
Overtime Hrs. per Week
Overtime Pay per Hour
Continue

Figure 133A

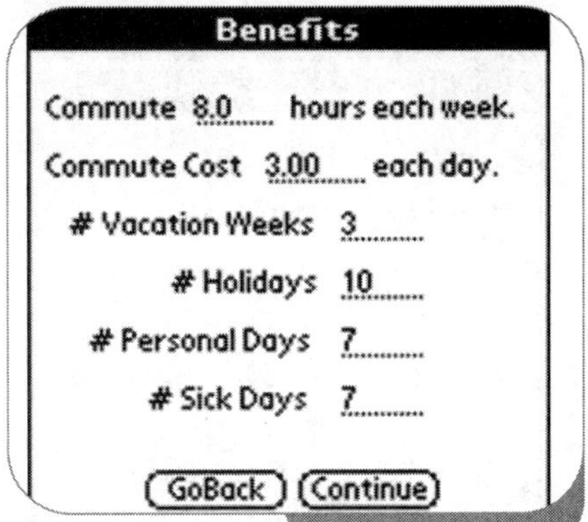
Benefits
Commute 8.0 hours each week.
Commute Cost 3.00 each day.
Vacation Weeks 3
Holidays 10
Personal Days 7
Sick Days 7
GoBack
Continue

Figure 133B

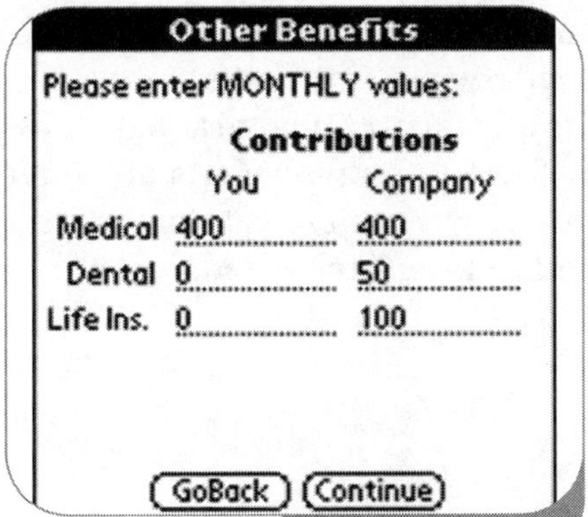
Other Benefits
Please enter MONTHLY values:
Contributions
You
Company
Medical 400 400
Dental 0 50
Life Ins. 0 100
GoBack
Continue

Figure 133C

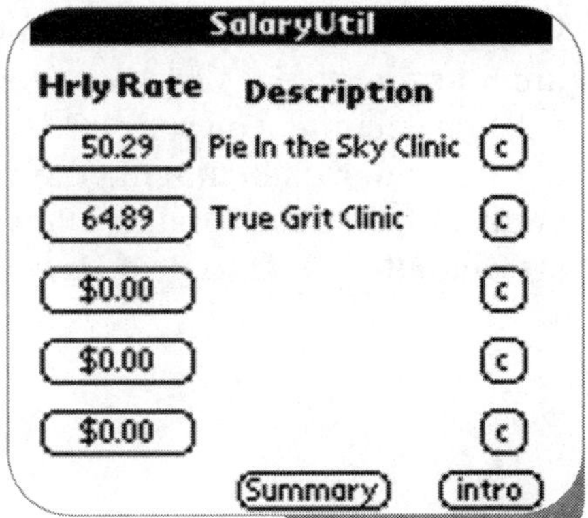

Figure 133D

function. When you do, you have a full-featured word processor at your fingertips immediately. It allows you to do the same kind of text formatting that you would expect to do on any other word processor. You can align text left, right, or center. You can make type bold, italic, strike through, or underlined. You can further choose one of four type sizes (superimposed on top of one of the other previously mentioned four choices) (Figure 134).

It gets better. You have the option to install one or a host of new typefaces to choose from, and Word Smith comes complete with thesaurus and spell checker built in. To my amazement, I also found that the latter two databases could operate just fine from my external memory. This frees up valuable internal memory on my PDA.

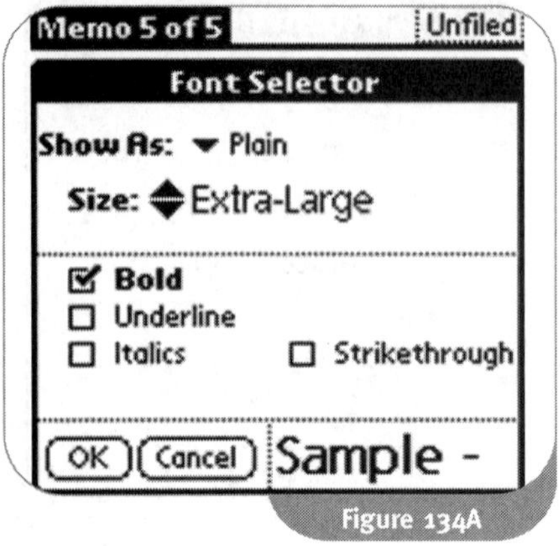

Figure 134A

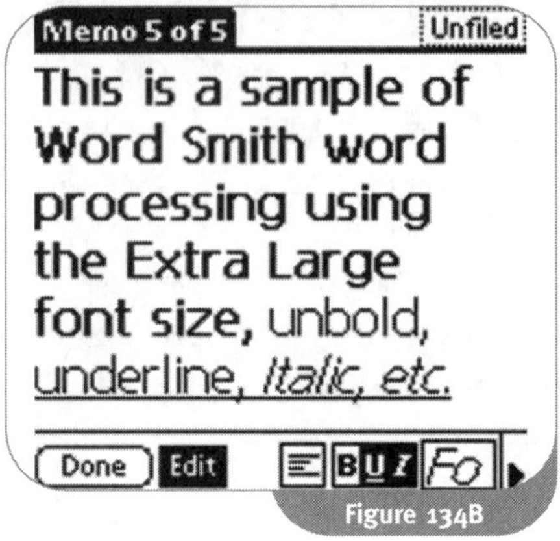

Figure 134B

When you HotSync your PDA to your PC, your nicely formatted document synchronizes with it to be printed or incorporated into a preexisting document on your PC. This is quite a useful program. It allows me to compose documents the way I want on my PDA. As an added bonus, I have found that it allows me to write memos to myself that are actually bolder and/or larger and thus easier to read.

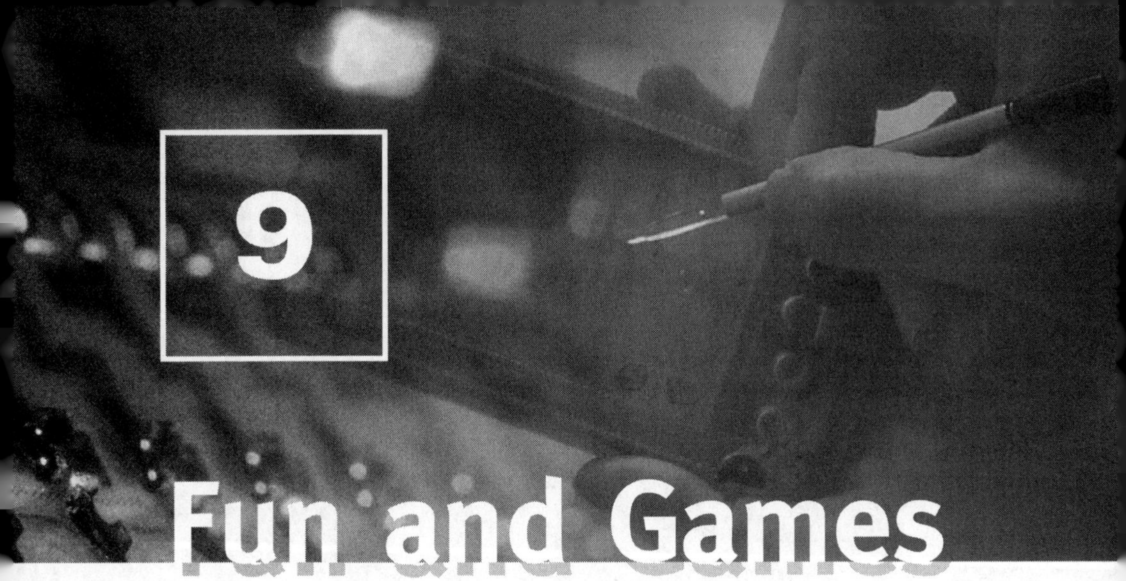

9 Fun and Games

Sometimes you just want to play and have fun, and sometimes you have time to kill (e.g., at the airport) and don't want to think or do anything particularly productive. Well, your PDA can hold many diversions, besides being such a productive tool. These diversions can amaze total strangers or can even be swapped with another user as you beam them back and forth.

Musical: Ebony Ivory, McChords, FretBoard, PocketSynth, Theremini

One of my favorite categories of diversions for the PDA is the music category. Although I am not a musician or a composer, few things evoke "I didn't know you could do that on one of those things" like pecking out a simple tune on a PDA piano keyboard. Ebony Ivory is just such a simple piano keyboard (Figure 135). Not only can you play tunes, it shows you the notation at the same time.

McChords takes this a step further. It identifies and plays the individual notes of a wide variety of chords (Figure 136). If you are more into the guitar, then FretBoard is the PDA equivalent because you can play guitar chords and scales on your PDA with it (Figure 137).

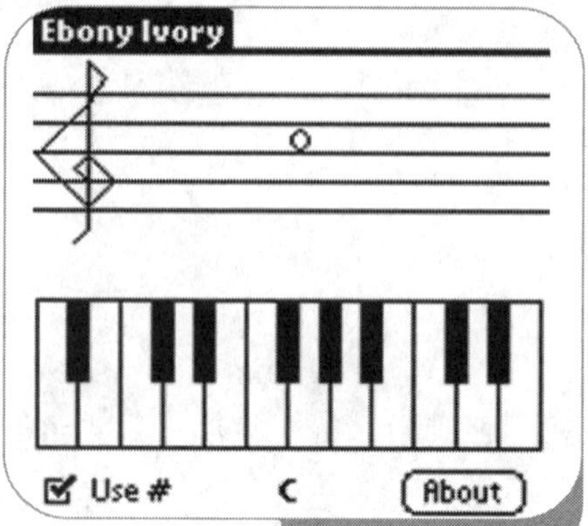

Figure 135

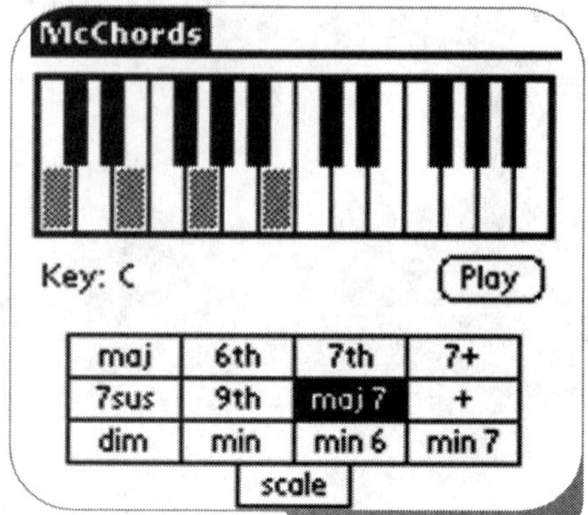

Figure 136

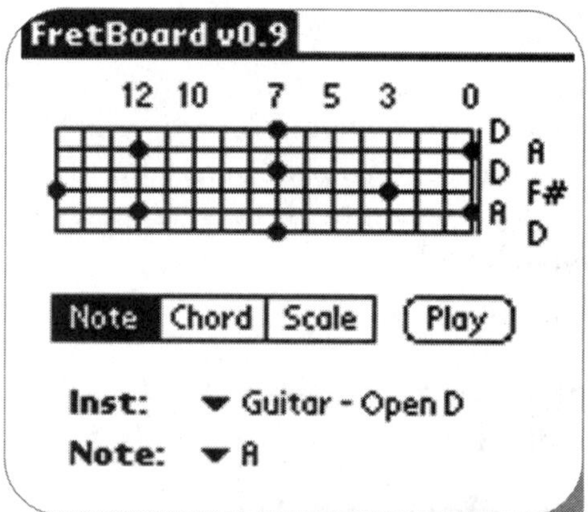

Figure 137

Finally, just for fun, there's Theremini, which is the PDA equivalent of the very first synthetic music instrument, the Theremin. You probably heard it in Sci-Fi movies of the 1950s. Now you can recreate those otherworldly sounds on your PDA by dragging the stylus across different parts of the screen, high-to-low to high again. You are in control of the sound. It is also a great way to annoy those around you.

Games: PocketChess, Pyramid, Yahdice, Invaders, etc.

So many games for the handheld computer exist that it would be easy to fill your entire memory with nothing but games. It is a vast category that has no end in sight. Clearly, a demand for games exists because the consuming public continues to buy them. I must admit that there are several to which I am addicted that help me to pass the time while waiting at the airport and other places. Some of the games are quite challenging, and some can be played against other players. Some are classic favorites such as board games, and some can even be played across the table with another PDA user by infrared beaming. Here are just a very few of the freeware/shareware offerings to whet your appetite. Many more commercial offerings are also available, with the list growing rapidly in this category.

PocketChess is a widely distributed electronic version of the classic board game. You play against the computer at any of various skill levels or play against a human opponent. The graphics are classically simple and straightforward. Good commands are available to the user, too. At my skill level, my favorite is the Undo command. I tell myself that I am actually teaching myself better chess when I take back a move (Figure 138).

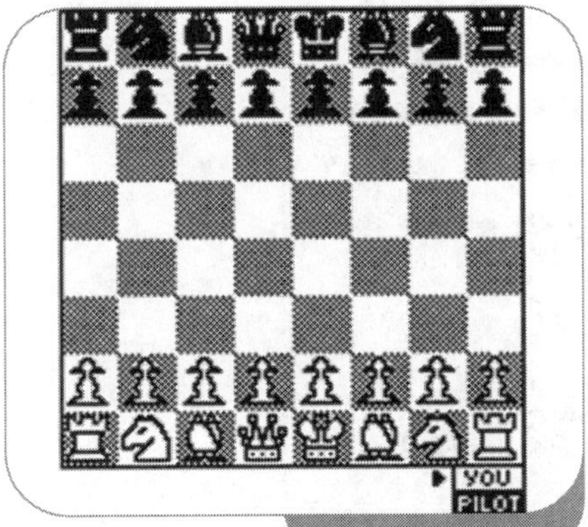

Figure 138A

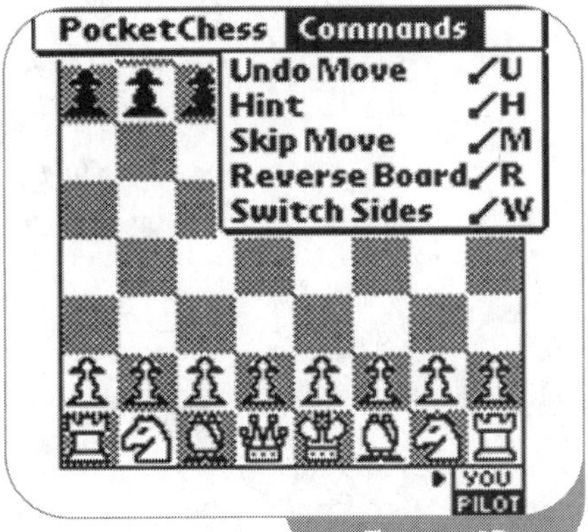

Figure 138B

Yahdice is the PDA equivalent of the classic dice game Yahtzee. You can play solitaire, just trying to increase your personal best, or play against other players. The game comes with fairly good instructions, is quick to play, and is truly addictive (Figure 139).

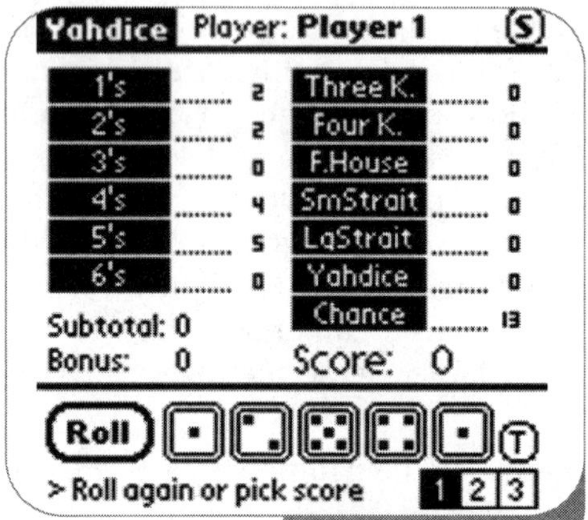
Yahdice
Player: Player 1
S
1's 2
2's 2
3's 0
4's 4
5's 5
6's 0
Three K. 0
Four K. 0
F.House 0
SmStrait 0
LgStrait 0
Yahdice 0
Chance 13
Subtotal: 0
Bonus: 0
Score: 0
Roll
T
> Roll again or pick score
1 2 3

Figure 139

If you're my age, you might remember the classic arcade game Space Invaders. Invaders is a nifty PDA version of this action shoot-em-up game. Frankly, I don't seem to have the coordination, dexterity, or eyesight to play this sort of game on my handheld. I include it here as a representative example of the type. Kids love it as it has lots of movement and takes up very little memory on your PDA (Figure 140).

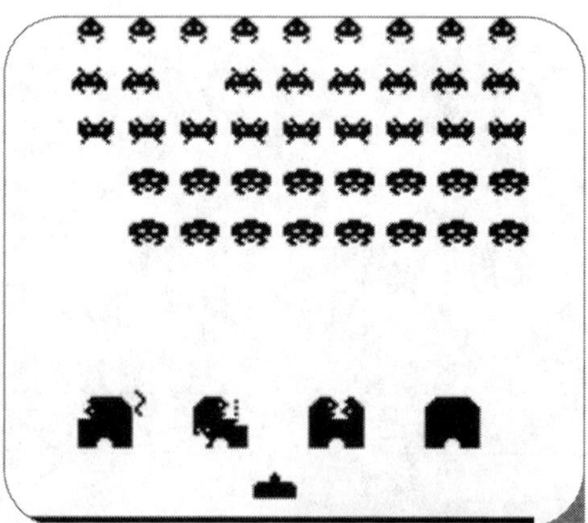

Figure 140

Planetarium

This really is an amazing program. If anybody ever doubts that a PDA is a real computer, just show him or her Planetarium (by Andreas Hofer, available at www.aho.ch/pilotplanets/release.htm). You input your own latitude and longitude, and this program charts the heavens for you. It does this graphically with an amazing number of stars, planets, and other objects that are customized for your locality and time. Planetarium can diagram the constellations for you. You can also tap on various items to have the program name them for you. Tap on a major (and often minor) star, and Planetarium will display its name. You can tap on a planet or constellation, similarly, and its name will pop up (Figure 141).

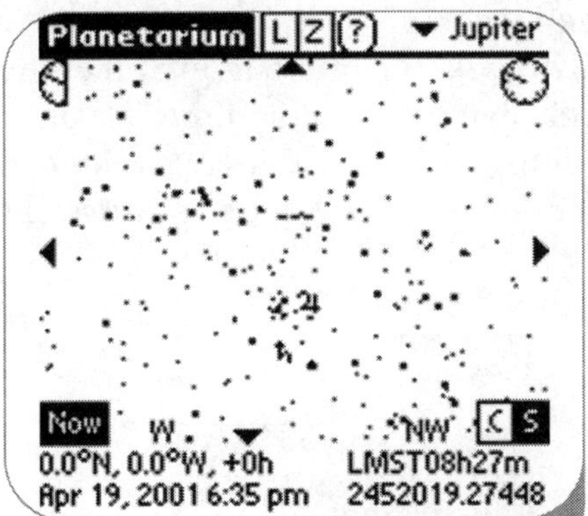

Figure 141A

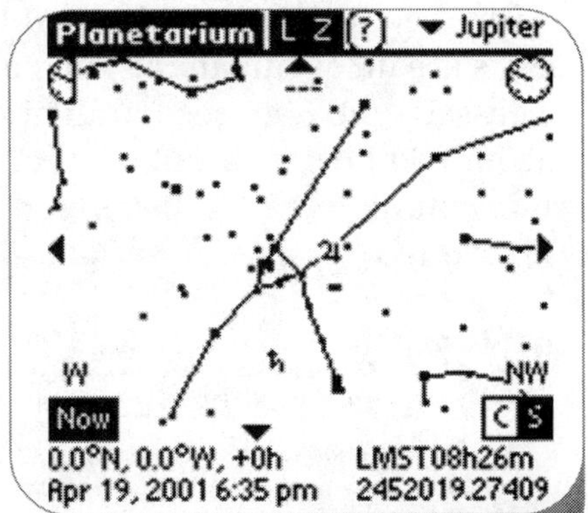

Figure 141B

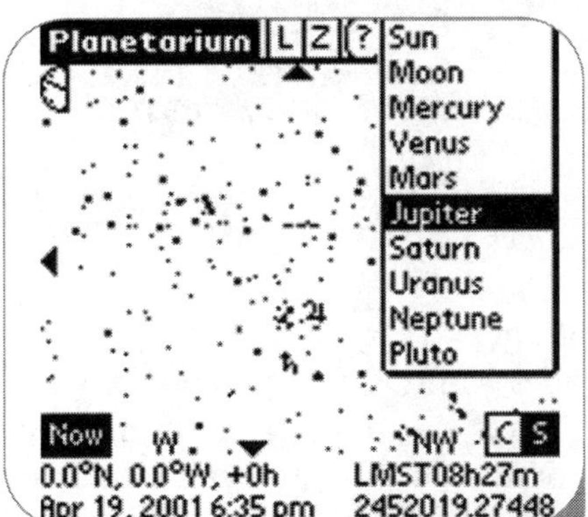

Figure 142A

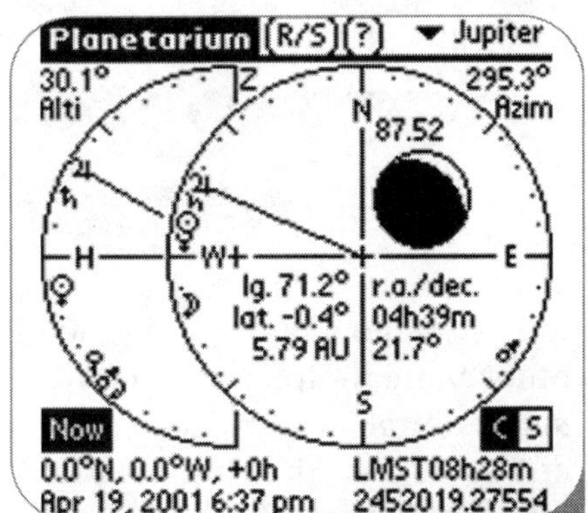

Figure 142B

Besides being a great way to show off the power of your PDA, Planetarium actually has practical uses. If you are into celestial navigation for your sailing adventures, you have probably already grasped the value of this program. It also includes instructions to make your PDA into an accurate compass. You can also change the display of Planetarium to reverse for backlighting and easier use when viewing the night sky (Figure 142).

DiveLog/DiveTable

Whatever your hobbies, handheld programs are available to assist you. If you happen to be a scuba diver, you are in luck. Here is a pair of handy dive programs.

DiveLog, logically, helps you keep track of your dives. The entry pages are nicely arranged and easily navigated and contain all of the necessary entry spaces for all of your dive data and comments. Once the individual dive is entered completely, it is automatically added to your cumulative dive list which can be sorted by geographic areas (Figure 143).

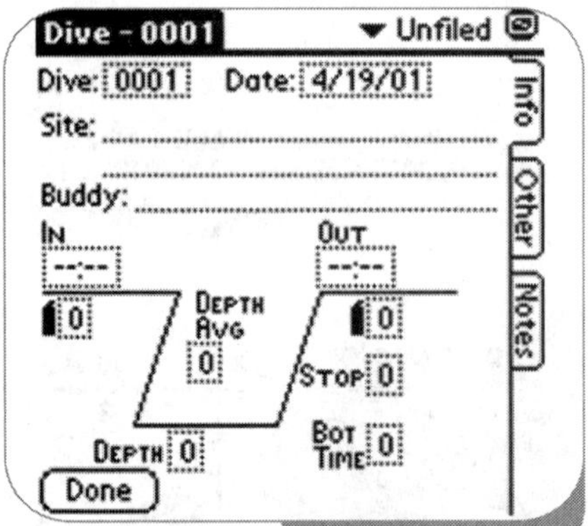

Figure 143A

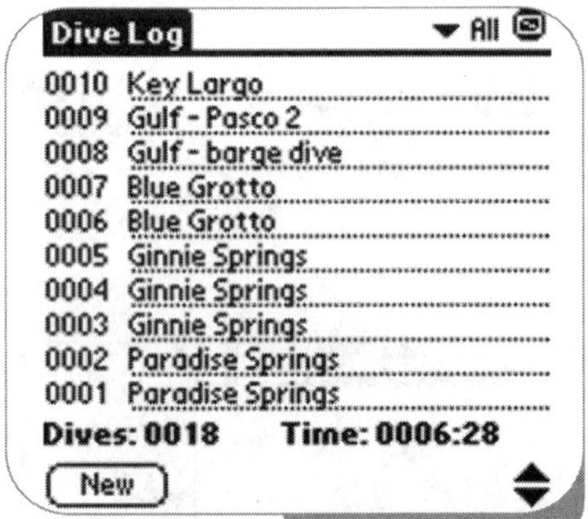

Dive Log
All
0010 Key Largo
0009 Gulf - Pasco 2
0008 Gulf - barge dive
0007 Blue Grotto
0006 Blue Grotto
0005 Ginnie Springs
0004 Ginnie Springs
0003 Ginnie Springs
0002 Paradise Springs
0001 Paradise Springs
Dives: 0018
Time: 0006:28
New

Figure 143B

DiveTable (by Bill Ezell, available at www.quackers.net), on the other hand, helps you to compute acceptably safe bottom times and surface times for repetitive dives. This is a simple graphic interface and you follow the charts, much as you would a printed version. If you already take your PDA with you on the boat, a printed dive table is just one less thing you now need to take with you (Figure 144).

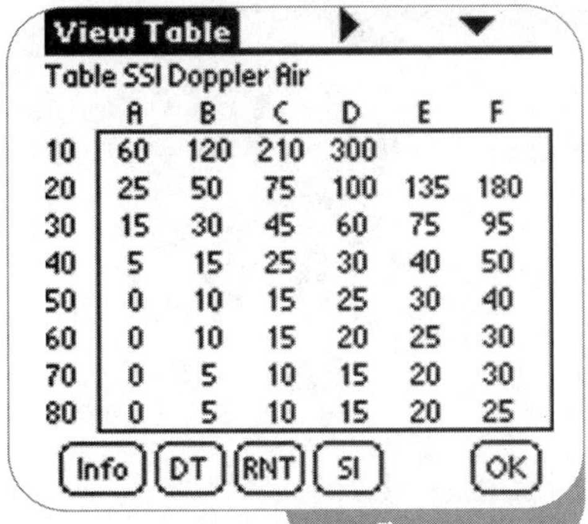

View Table

Table SSI Doppler Air

	A	B	C	D	E	F
10	60	120	210	300		
20	25	50	75	100	135	180
30	15	30	45	60	75	95
40	5	15	25	30	40	50
50	0	10	15	25	30	40
60	0	10	15	20	25	30
70	0	5	10	15	20	30
80	0	5	10	15	20	25

Figure 144

FlashBoom

This is one of the smallest of freeware programs (by Kim Moelgaard, available at http://home2.inet.tele.dk/kim_maj/flashboom.zip; also check out the author's Count It at http://home2.inet.tele.dk/kim_maj/), and it's just plain fun. Imagine the look on friends' faces when you tell them that with two touches of your PDA's stylus, you can tell how far away the next lightning strike occurs. You tap once when you see the flash and once when you hear the boom (hence FlashBoom), and the program calculates the distance. It has adorable graphics that visually depict the distance and can be calibrated to deliver answers in English or metric. This is just too awesome not to have (Figure 145)

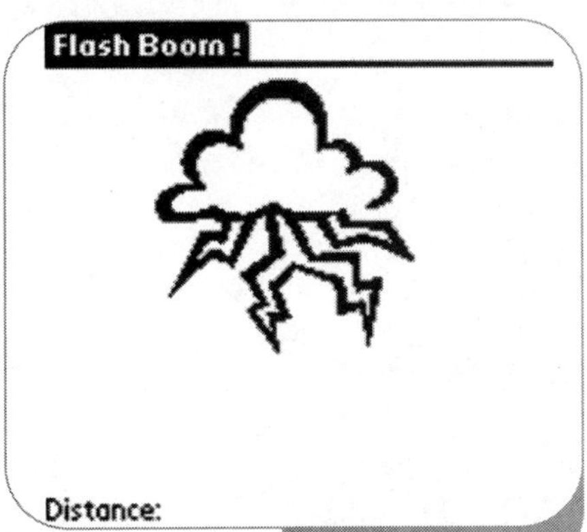

Figure 145A

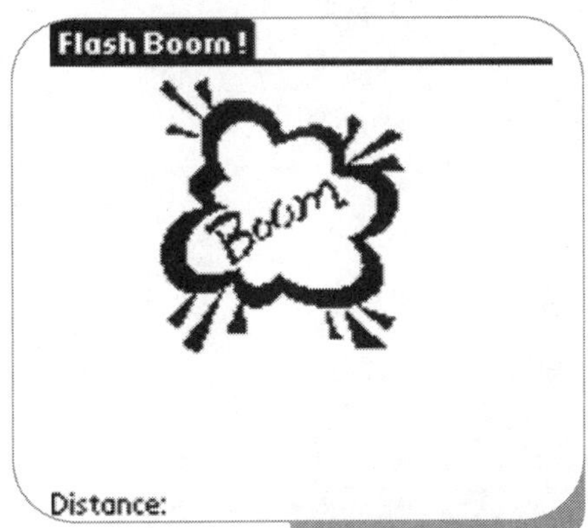

Figure 145B

Figure 145 Continued

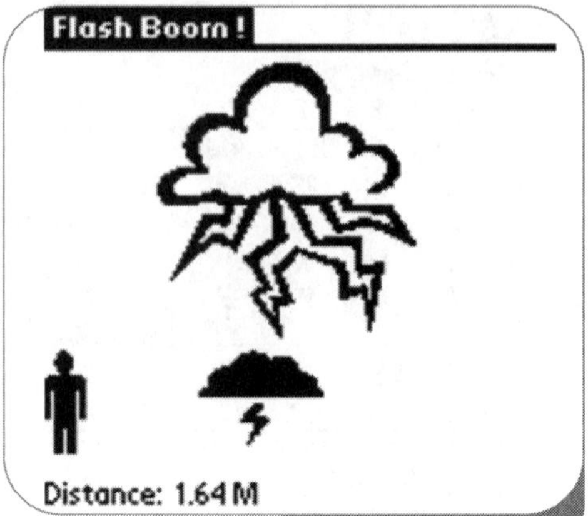

Figure 145C

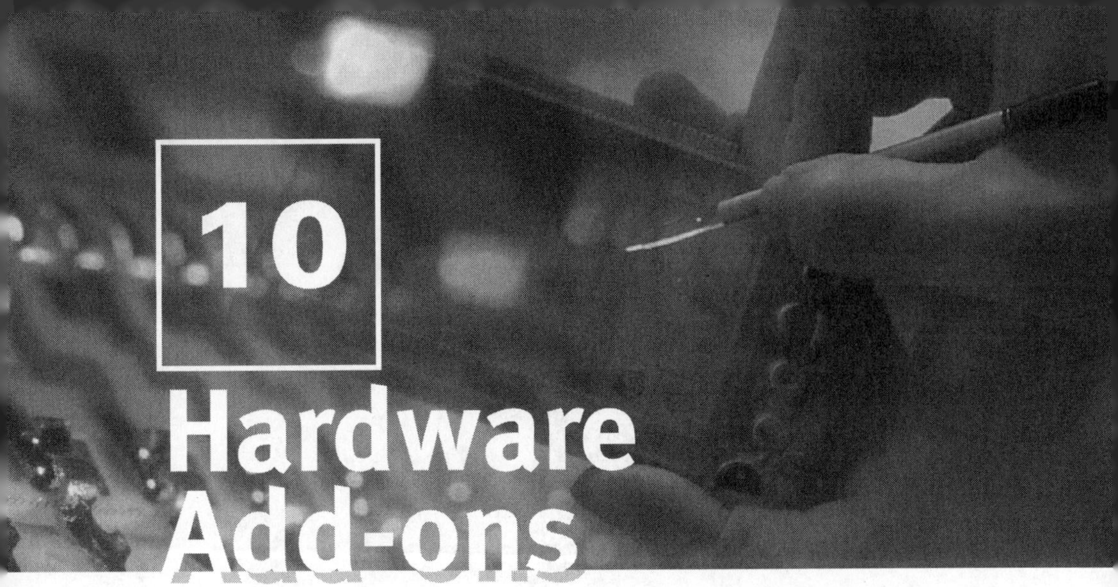

10 Hardware Add-ons

PDAs have advanced technologically and have many accessories that we can attach to them. A growing trend exists for manufacturers to equip handheld computers with more bells and whistles. However, with even the most stripped-down original purchase, wondrous aftermarket goodies are available for you to add. I am personally a "gadget freak," but that doesn't mean that I advocate buying all of the following attachments. You have to decide what is necessary, desirable, and affordable for you. Personal needs and tastes vary widely. Fortunately, manufacturers seem to cater to all of us.

Keyboards

Since I began research for this book, it seems that more PDA users have felt the need for some alternative to Graffiti for their data input. As a result, keyboards that were once available only as add-on devices to handheld computers have begun to give way to an assortment of built-in keyboard options. The impetus for this was probably the Research In Motion device called Blackberry. The Blackberry comes with a built-in "thumb" keyboard that lets the user input text messages with their two thumbs on a tiny keyboard. This idea has been reborn in such mainstream PDAs as the HandSpring Treo line and some of the Sony Clie models (Figure 146).

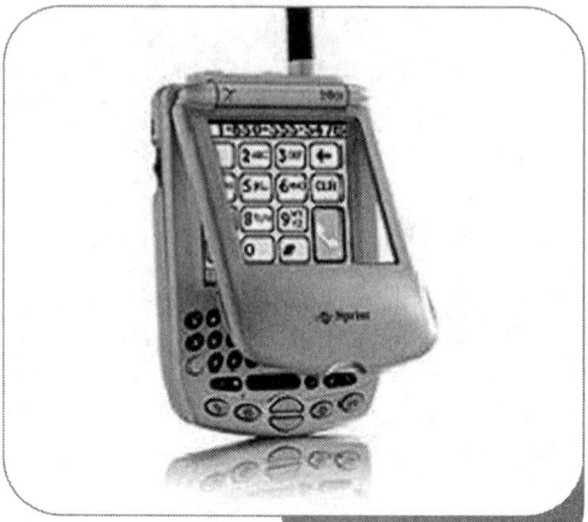

Figure 146A

Figure 146A (above) shows the built-in thumb keyboard peeking out from under the fliptop of one of the HandSpring Treo models. Figure 146B is the Sony Clie PEG-NX70 with a built-in thumb keyboard (the photo is courtesy of Sony Corporation of America).

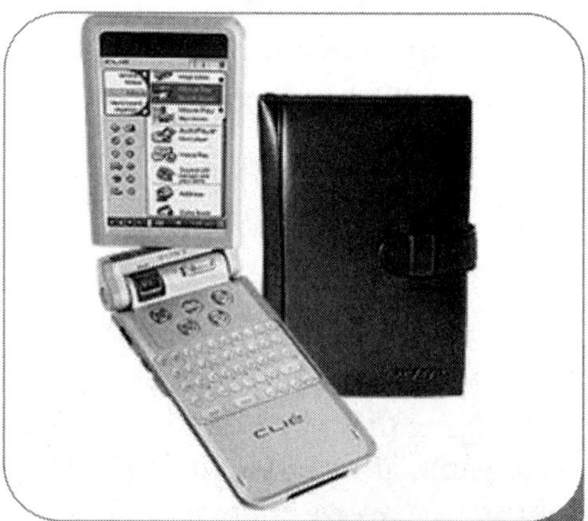

Figure 146B

If your PDA does not sport one of these built-in thumb keyboards, it is likely that you can add one from a number of different manufacturers. They now come in models to fit nearly every make and model of PDA. Although they may not be the ultimate answer for the input of large amounts of text data, many people find them a useful adjunct and often quite a bit faster than Graffiti input. I have one to add to my

HandSpring Visor Pro. It weighs next to nothing, hardly changes the profile of the PDA, and requires no separate battery because it draws its minimal power requirements directly from the PDA itself. I just pop it onto the bottom of my PDA and tap out text on its buttons. Figure 147 shows one of the Palm models with a typical thumb keyboard add-on.

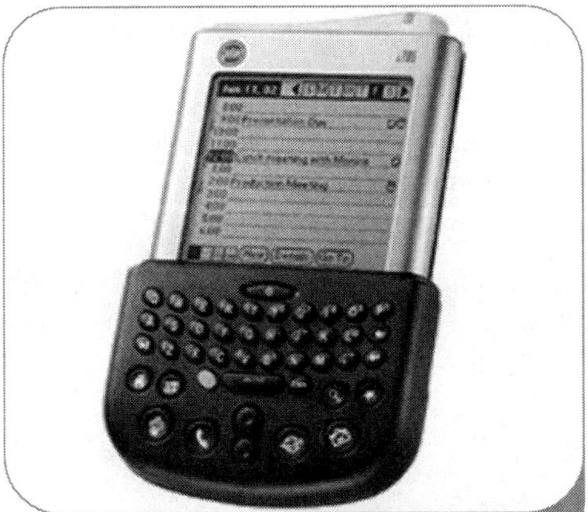

Figure 147

Probably the best solution for the input of large amounts of text data directly into a PDA is the add-on full-sized keyboard. Again, these are now available for nearly every make and model of handheld device. I use the Targus Stowaway Folding Keyboard (Figure 148). It folds up to about the same size as the PDA itself. When opened, it is a full-sized keyboard to which the PDA attaches easily. Once attached, the user just types away exactly as you would at a computer keyboard, but the results show up on your PDA's screen. As with the various thumb keyboards, the full-sized keyboard is powered directly by the PDA that is docked to it. The only drawback, aside from something extra to carry, is that the folding keyboards do require a flat firm surface for setup and use. You wouldn't want to try to operate one of them in your lap. However, you could easily operate the keyboard/PDA combination from an airplane tray table or at a nurse's station in a hospital.

I understand that there are actually full-size keyboards that communicate with the PDA wirelessly via the infrared beaming port. These

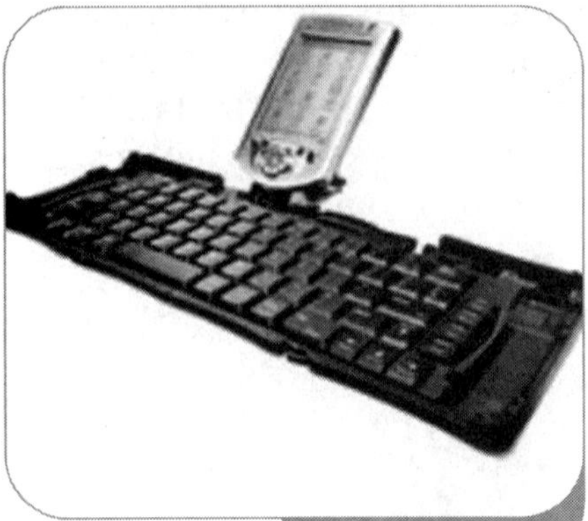

Figure 148A

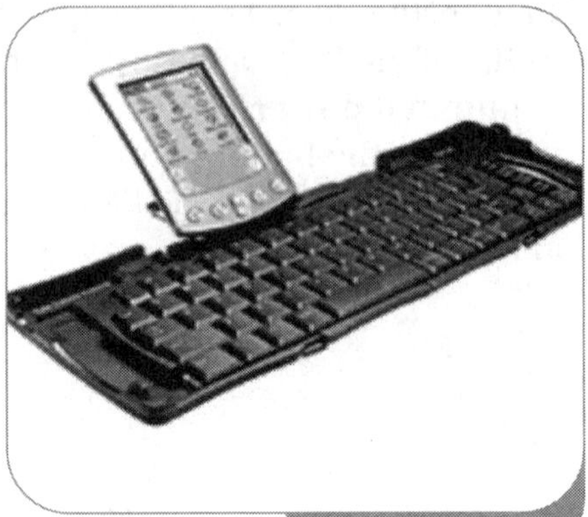

Figure 148B

keyboards free up the user from the necessity of physically docking the PDA to the keyboard. They would also presumably be more flexible in their ease of use.

Cameras

Certainly not every PDA user needs a camera as part of the device. However, for some users, a handy digital camera makes sense. As with the history of the keyboards illustrated previously here, these have begun to appear as built-in features of some models (most notably the Sony Clie PEG-NX70V model). Nevertheless, if yours does not have a built in digital camera, there's a good chance that there's an add-on camera available to fit your model. I use a Targus HandCam attached to my HandSpring Visor Pro. The memory expansion slots of many PDA models hold the promise of the possibility of camera add-ons in their futures if they are not currently available to fit.

Figure 149 shows one of the digital camera add-ons installed on one the HandSpring Visor models. The image on the screen was shot with the camera.

Thus far, none of these digital cameras are capable of stellar results because of inherently low resolution. If you're looking for images to rival 35 mm, you are in for some disappointment. However, what these cameras lack in image quality, they may make up for in convenience. After all, if you have one on your PDA and your PDA is always with you, then you always have a camera handy too. The im-

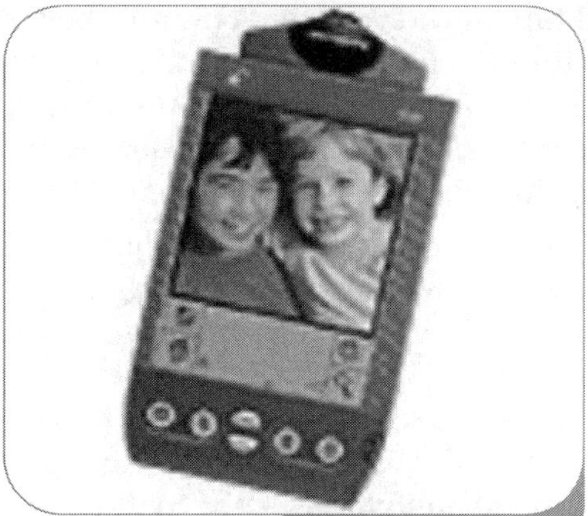

Figure 149

ages are fine for viewing in small format and can even be acceptable in small size on your PC. The bonus is that even if your PDA is a monochrome model, the cameras all shoot in color. This means that you can view the pictures later on your PC in color. Most of these cameras also come with a suite of software that allows you to use the pictures in ingenious ways. Some software, for example, allows you to place small snapshots right into appropriate places in your PDA's address book: put a face with that name. Other software actually allows the camera to be used to capture short minimovies.

None of this picture taking and movie making are without its cost to your PDA, however. You'd better plan to have plenty of available memory if you're going to capture and store any number of images. Luckily, you can usually move picture files over to external memory so that you can save them without occupying valuable internal memory space.

Phones

Probably the greatest buzz in the PDA world is the convergence of handheld technology with telephone technology. To me, this is so natural that it seems inevitable. Where previously I wore a cell phone on one hip and my PDA on the other, I now have them combined into one device. My phone benefits by having the brainier interface of an attached PDA. For example, I can look up a contact in my PDA's address book, and tap on the contact. The number is then automatically dialed into my attached cell phone. This so-called convergence technology seems to be the direction of the future. What you must decide is whether you need a PDA that is also a phone, or a phone that is also a PDA. Fortunately, the choices are becoming more numerous.

The HandSpring Treo line of PDAs seems one of the more successful marriages of PDA/phone technology. Certainly, it is not the only choice in this category, but it remains a good one. HandSpring has maintained all of the functionality of a PDA while incorporating a full-function cell phone in the same chassis. A flip-top design protects the built-in thumb keyboard while leaving the screen visible. Currently, two color models are available with built-in thumb keyboard, and one monochrome model has an option of built-in thumb keyboard or Graffiti area (Figure 150).

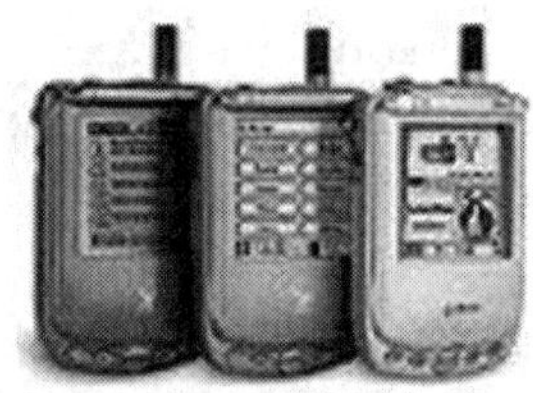

Figure 150

Other possibilities in this arena are available as well. Check out the convergence of PDA and phone technologies by Samsung (Figure 151A) or Kyocera (Figure 151B) as other options. Surely more are on the horizon, as this idea makes sense.

Another possibility is that a cell phone may be available as an add-on device to some selected PDA models. Is this reminiscent of keyboards and cameras (discussed previously)? I think so. In fact, I believe the add-on phone was available before the convergence models. Being habitually one step behind, I use an add-on phone module called the

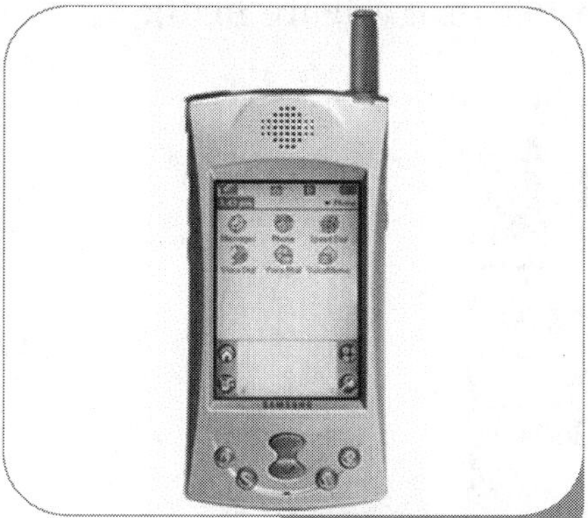

Figure 151A

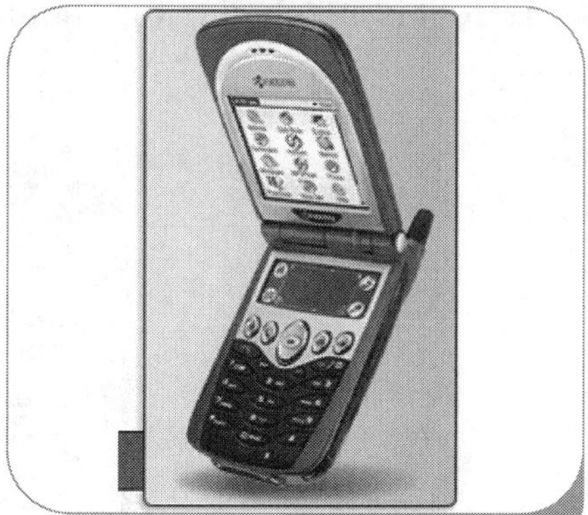

Figure 151B

VisorPhone on my HandSpring Visor Pro. It is a happy marriage of form and function and keeps me from carrying two separate devices. My VisorPhone is capable of doing all of the things that the convergence devices do, and my PDA is the same old functional device that it always was. In fact, I have the ability to pop out my phone module and pop in other expansion modules (e.g., expansion memory or the digital camera). This is something that the Treos can't yet do. I expect that to change soon with the advent of new models from HandSpring (Figure 152).

Here's the VisorPhone module (Figure 152A).

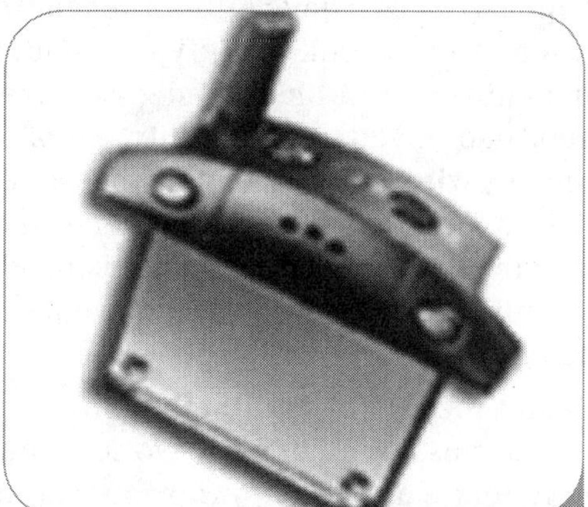

Figure 152A

Here it is attached to the HandSpring Visor (Figure 152B).

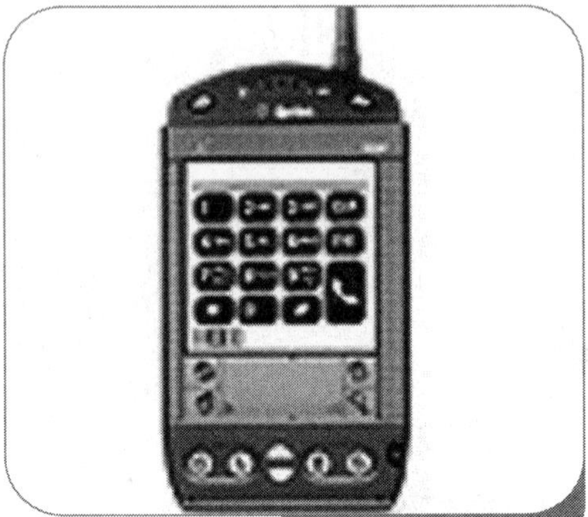

Figure 152B

Wireless Modems

I won't bore you with continuous pictures of hardware and hardware add-on possibilities, but a few categories still need to be mentioned. Wireless connectivity is one of these. Increasingly, PDA users seem to want to be able to access the Internet for a variety of purposes from checking their e-mail to "surfing the net" for more information and downloads. Although this capability comes at a price, it is increasingly available. Newer models such as the Palm Tungsten series or Sony Clie NX and NZ series have either the feature built in or have it available as an add-on. HandSpring Visor models have long had such modules available as add-ons. HandSpring Treo models that include cell phones also have this capability. All of these refer to the hardware that makes wireless connectivity possible. The other piece that you have to be aware of is that you would also have to subscribe to an Internet service that would work with your PDA. It is a combination deal. Monthly fees would apply, but the possibilities that this opens up are staggering.

Other makes and models of handheld computers may also have wireless connectivity possibilities. Some work in conjunction with the proper model cell phone and the appropriate connector cord. Many models of Pocket PC devices also have wireless connectivity possibilities. Just check with your manufacturer's web site.

MP-3 Players

If you are a music fan, you may want to carry this type of diversion in your PDA. As with the previously mentioned category, newer models (again, notably the Palm Tungsten series and Sony Clie NX and NZ series) come with this feature built in. Other models increasingly have MP3 capability available as an add-on feature. You capture, convert, or record music in the MP3 format and store it digitally in the PDA's external memory storage card. Generally, playback is through earphones for very good quality sound. This makes your PDA a very handy personal entertainment center.

Voice Recorders

At the risk of becoming repetitive, this PDA product category is much like the last two. Handheld users began early on to enjoy the possibilities of a device that included voice recording among its bag of tricks. Pocket PC models were probably the first to incorporate this feature, but the Palm OS devices have been quickly catching up. First available as add-on modules to the HandSpring Visor line, voice recording now comes as a standard built-in feature on the latest models like the Palm Tungsten series and the Sony Clie NX and NZ series. Always with you and ever handy for quick reminders, voice recordings can also be creatively appended to e-mails or other files, swapped, beamed, or downloaded to your PC in many cases. Again, the possibilities are unlimited.

GPS Receivers

For those of you that don't know, GPS stands for Global Positioning Satellite, the marvelous marriage of land-based and space technology that can pinpoint any location on earth to within a few feet. If you have a GPS receiver and the right software, you are in communication with a network of satellites that are in Earth orbit, and you use this connection for navigation purposes. This is the technology behind the installations in upscale cars that tell the driver where they are, where they are going, and how to get there turn by turn in real time.

In the past, you might add the software/hardware combination to acquire GPS capability to a laptop computer. Now, with a growing number of add-on modules, you can add a GPS to many PDAs. HandSpring Visors have this capability, although you would have to check other makes and models specifically for available add-ons. Garmin, a long-time maker of stand-alone GPS receivers and software, has recently announced that it will offer a PDA, using Palm OS, which will have a built-in GPS.

Presenter To Go

This is one of my favorite hardware/software add-ons (by Margi), and it seems to be little known among PDA users. Imagine that you are a speaker at an upcoming conference. Furthermore, you have prepared an elegant PowerPoint presentation in lieu of the old-fashioned and accident-prone slide presentation. You could lug around a laptop computer to attach to the LCD projector at the conference. Instead, you could install the whole PowerPoint presentation to your PDA with the Presenter To Go software, carry your presentation in your PDA, attach the PDA directly to the LCD projector with the supplied hardware and cord, and present directly from your PDA. People will be amazed! Leave the laptop at home. A tiny wireless remote even exists to advance the "slides," go back, etc. You can view speaker notes on your PDA as you speak, too (Figure 153).

Figure 153 shows the Margi Presenter To Go attaching a PDA to an LCD projector.

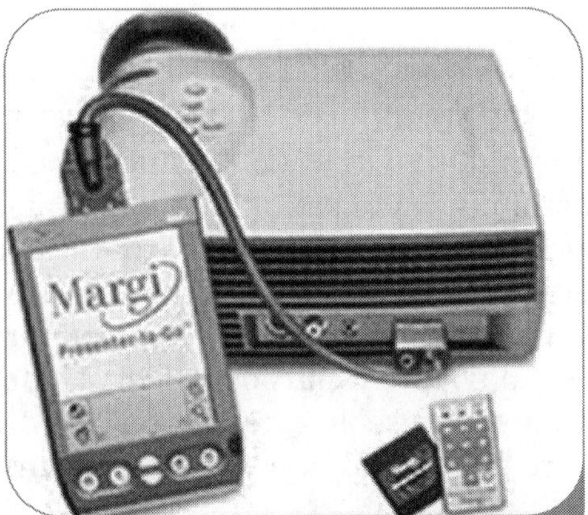

Figure 153

I find one more piece of the software amazing and, frankly, it is the reason that I purchased Presenter To Go in the first place. That is Presenter To Go's ability to project PDA functions directly to the screen in real time. What does this mean? In my work teaching in a physician assistant program, I frequently want to show the students how to do something on their PDAs. How can one demonstrate something on their PDA except by having the other person look over your shoulder? Presenter To Go comes to the rescue. I merely slip the PTG module into the memory slot of the PDA, attach the power plug (preventing additional drain on the PDA's internal batteries), and attach the supplied cord directly to the LCD projector. With this, I can demonstrate most anything I do on the PDA to a large or small audience by projecting it on the screen.

Presenter To Go comes with additional memory built in to its memory plug-in. This means that you can often carry your presentation with you without taking up internal memory space in your PDA. My wish list would include Presenter To Go with even more external memory for larger presentations, but you will find that this suits most purposes right now. The Margi folks have accommodated many makes and models. Check their web site for availability for your particular model. Recently, I have begun to see Margi's Presenter To Go included with a free PDA with the purchase of a particular LCD projector. Considering the price tag of some of the LCD projectors, I think this is an excellent incentive and has me nearly salivating at the prospect (is my wife reading this?).

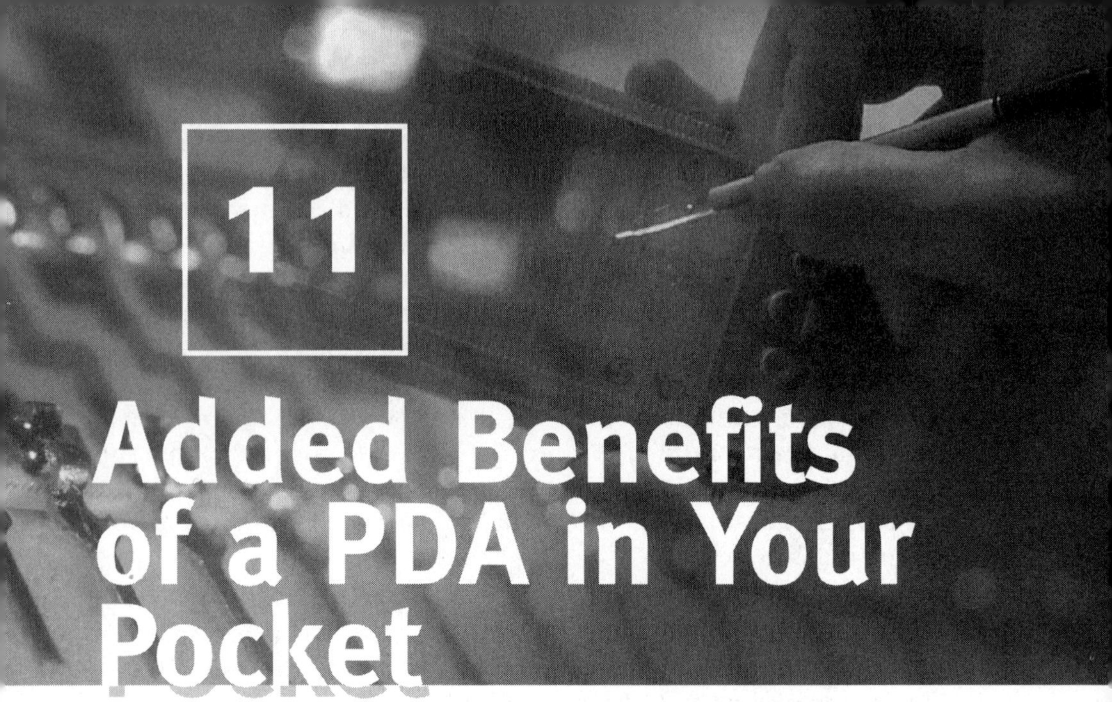

11 Added Benefits of a PDA in Your Pocket

Sometimes, refreshingly enough, you get more than you bargained for. Of course, you likely have some specific goals of what you want your handheld computer to accomplish for you. You may want it because it will help you organize your life, remember details, remind you of appointments, or serve as a great reference library. The amazing thing is that your PDA can do all of that and more. It still constantly surprises me with all of the bonus things I have learned from it in the process of using it daily.

Learning the Technology

For me, the most tangible side benefit of adopting a PDA into your daily life is learning and becoming comfortable with handheld technology itself. This is something that I try to express to students as well. Most students embrace this concept and are ahead of me. A few actually resist change, including technology. For the most part, however, most medical professionals recognize that change in medicine is ongoing. They also recognize that medicine is generally on the cutting edge of technology. Therefore, it makes sense that medical professionals would find a niche for PDAs in their practices. The more we use these tools, the more familiar we become with their features, their capabilities, and their potential.

This is probably why every PDA owner you talk to owns the "best" brand out there with the "best" features in the world. He or she probably bought it at the most amazing price, too. Besides post-purchase reinforcement, the fact is that we each become most comfortable with whatever it is that we are most familiar. Thus, I generally know the features of my Handspring Visor or my Sony Clie much better than I know those of any other brand of PDA. I can see advantages, even envy, the features of some other PDAs, but I will not be as familiar or as knowledgeable about them because I don't use them every day. Just having and using a handheld computer every day has much of the same sort of advantage inherent in it. The observer to this entire process might envision that a PDA could be a useful adjunct to his practice, but he or she would have no idea just how useful until he or she already owned one and began using it all of the time. Familiarity with the technology will come with regular use. I hope that with this book I have given you some quick-start guides to get you going. Daily use will get you through the rest because PDA use is quite intuitive. The rough spots are really those unplanned events and catastrophes (e.g., crashes). That is when you rely on in-depth instruction manuals and experienced good friends.

I tell students to treat their PDAs with the respect that computers deserve (not getting them wet, not dropping them, not scratching their screens, etc.); however, harm doesn't come from simply trying new things. The handheld computer is a friendly learning laboratory and is actually difficult to mess up. Of course, you should back it up frequently to your PC just in case. You are free to change your PDA's settings, its sounds, its categories, its display, and a host of other possibilities. Experiment. Explore. Push buttons. Try things out. That's the fun of owning a PDA! Soon, you will be showing others about your new discoveries and helping them to get started.

ICD Coding

Medicine has become increasingly complex. Of this, there is no doubt. Therefore, anything that brings a measure of standardization and organization to medicine strikes me as a good thing. Such is the basic case for ICD coding. Unfortunately, few of us currently practicing medicine were taught much about ICD coding, nor are we very familiar with it. ICD coding is often left up to the front office staff of a given medical practice. It's too bad because clinicians are the ones most likely to have a better technical grasp of the medical diagnoses involved. The good news is that with a little use of the PDA incorporated into daily practice, clinicians can painlessly become more familiar with the ICD codes used in their practice. I see this as a side benefit. You didn't set out to learn those codes. You didn't purchase a set of flash cards to learn them. Nevertheless, with daily use, they become part of your knowledge base.

How does this happen? It can happen via patient tracking. If you use your PDA for patient tracking functions (keeping some sort of patient notes in your handheld), then you likely have ICD codes built into your patient tracking software. As you enter a patient into the database of your PDA, you will also be assigning an ICD code to that patient. As you do this repeatedly, you will be learning about some of your most frequently used ICD codes. You might occasionally even want to sort your patient encounters by ICD code just to look at this particular category.

This is exactly what has happened to our students. We require them to log their clinical encounters, including the ICD codes. In the process, they have learned far more about common ICD codes than they would have just by reading about them. Some of our students have even taken the initiative to add to the ICD code database when they found themselves in a clinical specialty that used different codes than the basic database included.

DSM Coding

The added benefit of learning DSM codes in a psychiatric setting is similar to the argument mentioned previously. Several good programs for the PDA (some of them free) provide quick and accurate DSM codes for psychiatric diagnoses. Having such a reference in your PDA, if you're in such a practice, makes good sense. As you use them, you will learn them. For those that you use infrequently, well, that's why you have a reference in your pocket.

CPT Coding

For surgical procedures, CPT coding brings the same organization and uniformity to medicine as the ICD codes do to diagnoses. The PDA user has the same potential for secondary gain of knowledge by using a CPT code database in daily practice, and these, too, are available.

Billing and Coding

In the area of evaluation and management coding, many practices actually do a poor job. Much like ICD coding, clinicians have generally been insufficiently trained in this area and have therefore left this responsibility to the front office staff. Many practices routinely undercode for fear of being audited and having fines that result from overcoding. This means lost revenue to the practice. This need not be the case with the incorporation of one of the several fine evaluation and management coding software programs available for the PDA. A clinician who spends a few minutes incorporating evaluation and management coding into his or her daily routine will be rewarded by a better understanding of the coding process, more income for the practice, and probably more thorough exams as well.

Publication Downloads

Some regular medical publications such as *The Prescriber's Letter*, *The Medical Letter*, and *The New England Journal of Medicine*, recognizing the proliferation of PDAs in medicine, now offer PDA downloads as a regular feature to their subscribers. Not only can individual issues be downloaded to the PDA to read and reference on the road, but also bonus features such as *The Prescriber's Letter* Detail Documents are available in the PDA format. I look for more of this to follow from other publishers, as well. *The Prescriber's Letter* also has patient handouts that are available in PDA format. I can see increasing potential in beaming such documents to the right patients who just happen to own PDAs too. I think that patients would remember such practitioners in a much more favorable light.

Conference Downloads

To me, conference coordination and PDA downloads connected with conferences are the neatest thing seen in a while. You go to a medical conference armed with your PDA and get downloads associated with that conference, maybe programs that you can use later, or electronic conference materials that you can carry with you in your PDA. Would you buy a handheld computer just for this purpose? Probably not, so that's why it's in this chapter of added benefits to owning and using a PDA.

In September, 2002, the 52nd Annual Congress of Neurological Surgeons held "the first ever digital medical conference." They distributed 2,400 Palm i705 wireless PDAs to conference attendees. The devices reportedly came preinstalled with the complete meeting program, abstracts, graphs, x-rays, convention center and exhibit hall guide, hyperlinks to exhibitor information, Philadelphia city guide, and a complete membership directory. CNS President, Stephen M. Papadopoulos, M.D., was quoted as saying, "This large-scale digital effort is not just another medical meeting with computers. It represents a major paradigm shift in the way we will practice neurosurgery. Members and residents will participate in the meeting with the assistance of a Palm handheld that will educate, organize and simplify their complex practices."[1]

This is an exciting prospect. I expect that many more conferences will employ similar strategies to lure attendees. At the very least, you could anticipate increased offerings for PDAs at conferences. At the past few I have attended, PDA software vendors have certainly been in attendance who were glad to beam me trial versions of their software. I don't think I'll be attending any more conferences without my PDA handy.

[1] "Congress of Neurological Surgeons Holds First Digital Medical Conference Using Handheld Technologies." Internet article posted 9/26/2002 at PDA Cortex (www.rnPalm.com/cns.htm).

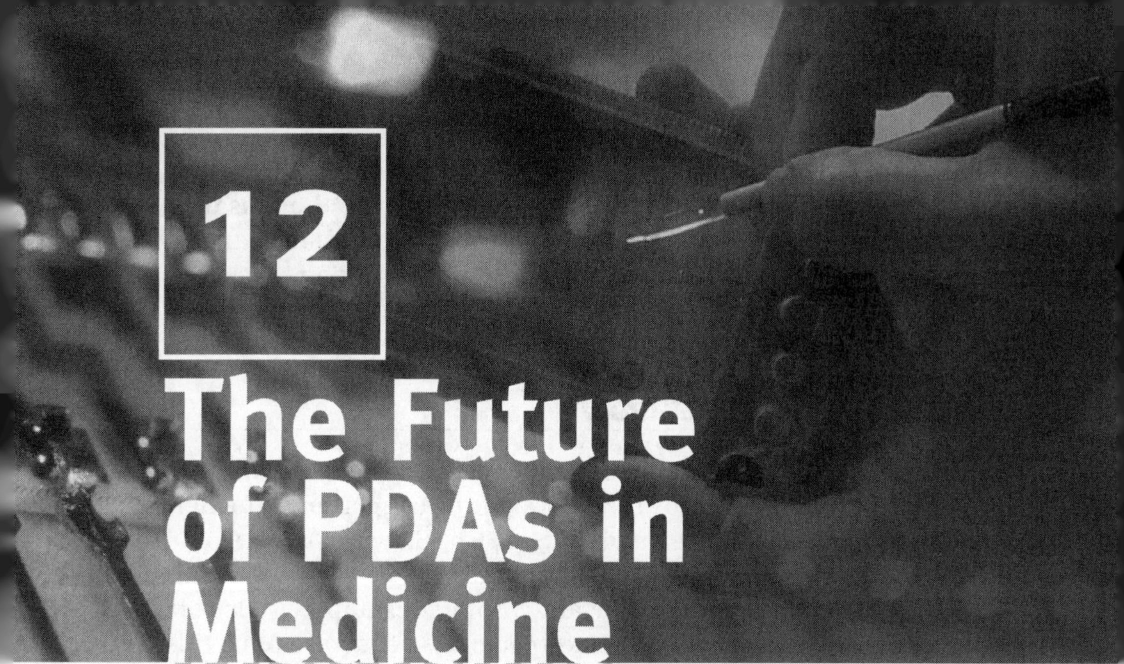

12 The Future of PDAs in Medicine

Here is where I get to have a little fun by getting out my crystal ball and trying to predict the future. You may not want to pay too much attention, however, as I didn't do too well in predicting the stock market. Based on what I've seen of PDAs and medicine in the past few years, significant reading, Internet browsing, and chatting with others about the subject, this is what I see for the future of these marvelous medical tools. As we see more medical professionals adopt the devices, more software being developed for medical purposes, and better and faster hardware, we should also see the following.

More Wireless: Prescribing, etc.

I believe that the price for Internet service will drop and that there will be more shared networks. This will make wireless Internet access into a more realistic and affordable venture for an increasing number of PDA users. The technology is already here. Sony's latest NX series of Clies has the ability to add WiFi cards for wireless access. Palm's Tungsten comes equipped with a BlueTooth wireless chip that will allow it to communicate wirelessly with similarly BlueTooth equipped devices (office PCs, cell phones, printers, etc.). The possibilities are endless. Some systems already use this wireless capability to allow a clinician to write prescriptions on his or her PDA and wirelessly transmit them to an office printer or computer to generate a written prescription that the patient would take with them as they leave the office. Increasingly, we will see systems that transmit directly from the office to the receiving pharmacy downstairs or across town.

Voice Recognition: Dictation

Clinicians have dictated their chart notes into voice recorders for years. Some PDAs have already incorporated voice recording into their hardware (e.g., Palm Tungsten and the Sony Clie SX series). You would not need to carry a separate voice recorder to complete the job. Voice recognition can't be far away. Certainly, some desktop PCs already can make use of some very good voice-recognition software. With this software, the user just speaks into a microphone, and the computer translates the spoken word into typed copy. No more transcription. Imagine this same capability in your PDA. I can and do.

More Multifunction

We have seen the proliferation of add-on modules with the Hand-Spring Visor line of PDAs. Multitudes of other add-ons are available for other brands of PDAs as well. It is a matter of supply and demand. If the consuming public wants multifunction devices, then the manufacturers will develop them. If we want more functions built in, then they will build them. It will be interesting to watch the trends in PDA/cell phone combinations. Voice recording, cameras, and more are already coming built in. The latest Sony Clie SX series even has infrared television remote control software built in to the device. My dream machine? Why not build a TV receiver right into the PDA? Talk about a multipurpose device!

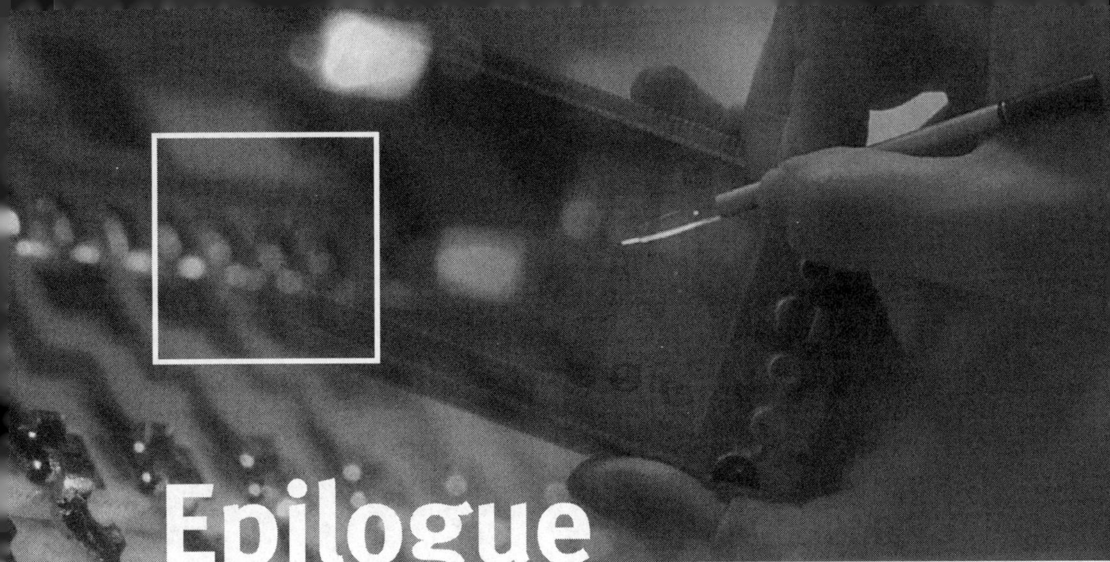

Epilogue

This is a book by a medical professional for other medical professionals. We have a long tradition of sharing with one another our successes and our failures and what we have learned from other colleagues. This book is in that tradition. I hope you will not only share with your colleagues but share your experiences with me as well, as I'm not infallible. Perhaps you could help me avoid making errors in future editions. Moreover, handheld computer technology, like medicine itself, is constantly changing. If the reader comes across something new and/or better, why not share it with all of us? If you have come across PDA software or hardware that you have found helpful (especially helpful in medicine), please let me know about it. It may have been overlooked or was too new to make it into this edition. If I have made an error, please let me know, as I welcome your feedback, comments, and suggestions. Feel free to contact me by e-mail at: chelopoulos@mail.barry.edu. Who knows, your name may actually appear in print in the next edition.

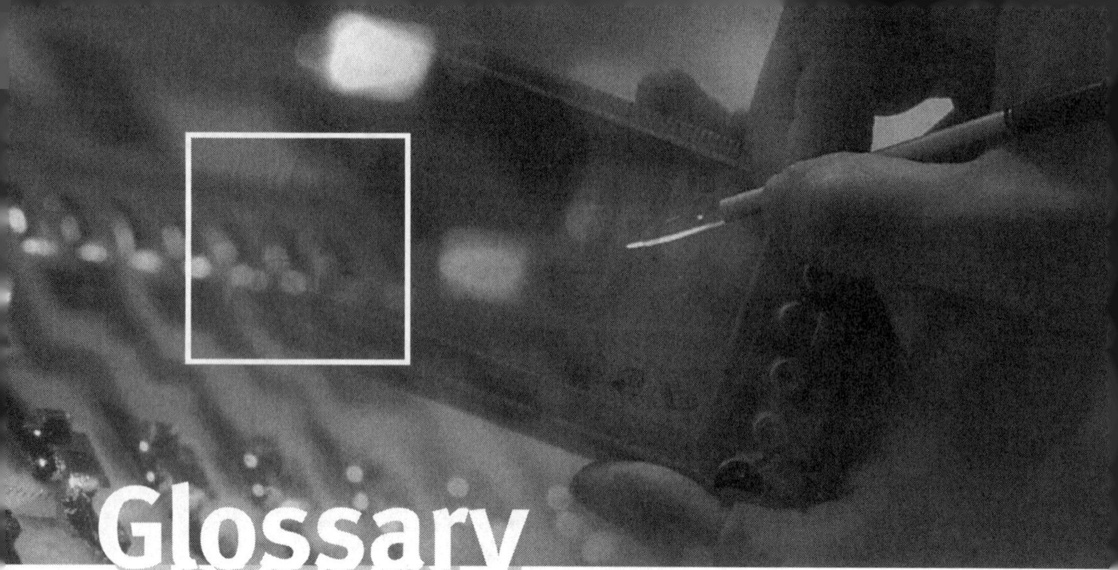

Glossary

These are my own definitions. I did not look them up; thus, they are my own interpretations, designed to help the novice get through this book more easily.

Applet—A software application-ette or subprogram. For example, Alticopeia is an applet that works within the HanDbase application. You must have HanDbase installed in your PDA to enable you to run Alticopeia. Applets are usually cheaper or free. Once you have an application, you might naturally want to see what applets are available for it.

Application—A software program that gives your PDA extra functionality.

Beam—To send data or applications wirelessly from one PDA to another using the built-in infrared transmitter/receiver. This works like the remote control for your TV. In fact, your PDA could become your TV/VCR remote control with the right software. Beaming also works between your PDA and suitably enabled printers, laptops, and other hardware.

Book mark—A feature that allows the reader of a PDA text to come back to a frequently used area repeatedly. The user sets the book marks and can later jump directly to any bookmarked spot.

CD-ROM—This is the acronym for Compact Disc-Read Only Memory. These are the familiar discs that you insert into your desktop computer or your audio CD player. They have programming (or music) written to them as a storage device. As they pertain to PDAs, these discs are the format of choice for the retailing of software for your PDA. If you went to an electronics store, this is how you would find PDA software on the shelf. You take it home, insert the disc in your desktop computer, follow the instructions, and then HotSync your PDA. I prefer this format because you always have a backup available by reinserting the original disc.

Crash—The much-feared loss of all of your PDA data. A crash usually involves having to reinstate your PDA to its original factory-issued condition. You will lose all data and any programs that you have added since the purchase. This is why you should back up your data and programs frequently by using HotSync.

Cursor—A small flashing bar on the screen of your PDA that indicates where an entry is about to be made. This is the marker of your data entry.

Demo/Trial Version (of software)—A version of software (application or applet) that is often free. It may be an abbreviated version of the full program, a trial version that is usable for a limited time, have a smaller capacity than the full version, or have built-in delays that remind you to pay for the full version.

Files (.pdb, .prc, etc.)—Different programs and bits of data for your PDA are stored in files on your PDA. This enables you to find, share, and move them around (e.g., to external memory cards). Different kinds of files have different suffixes. For example, files that end in .pdb are Palm Data Base files (that can usually be freely accessed from external memory cards). Files that end in .prc, on the other hand, are application files that usually must be stored in your PDA's internal memory.

Freeware—Software much like "shareware," but offered by the developer completely free with no expectation of a fee. This sounds too good to be true, but some developers just like to share, gain experience, and collect feedback from users.

Graffiti—This is the stylized printing that PDA users use to enter handwritten data into their handheld computers. The term is trademarked by Palm, Inc., and the Graffiti alphabet is used in all of the PDAs that use Palm OS. Graffiti enables the PDA to recognize exactly what the user is writing. It is typically entered in the designated Graffiti area of the PDA screen.

Hacks—These are small programs or applets called file extensions. Installed to your PDA with the appropriate hack enabler (HackMaster, TealMaster, etc.), a hack can squeeze extra versatility from your standard PDA applications.

HotSync—The means of communication and connectivity between your handheld computer and your regular computer. Usually this is accomplished by placing the handheld in a cradle that is connected by wire to your computer. This enables one- or two-way exchange of information. It is also the way that programs are installed in your handheld and the way that you automatically back up your data and programs. The term is trademarked by Palm, Inc., but the process is used by all of PDA brands that use Palm OS. A similar action is performed for Pocket PC devices as well.

Icon—A recognition symbol. Each of the software programs that you install to your PDA comes with its own icon so that you can easily spot the program on your PDA's launch screen.

Launch Button—On most PDA models this is the "silkscreen" button in the lower left-hand corner of the screen. It is the button that you tap to go to your launch screen. There you will see the icons or the list of all of the programs that you have installed on your PDA.

Locked Programs—These are registered, copyrighted commercial software that you had to pay for in order to use. If you try to beam one of these to another PDA user, you will see a small lock icon next to the program title and will receive a message reminding you that it will be impossible for you to beam this program.

Nag—Any of several types of pesky reminders that you haven't yet paid for that shareware. These may take the form of a reminder screen that you just have to tap on to remove, a countdown timer (delay), or others. The idea is to "guilt" you into registering and paying for the shareware, at which time the "nag" will go away.

OS or Operating System—This is language that your PDA operates with—its life blood. Practically speaking, there are two main camps: Palm OS (used by Palm, HandSpring, Sony, and HandEra brands) and Pocket PC (the Microsoft OS used by Casio, Compaq, Dell, and others). A few other minor players and brands exist. This book is largely concerned with Palm OS (as explained in the early chapters). Beware of organizers that use neither of these operating systems. Generally, one operating system is not compatible with another. Software generally comes in both types if you buy it as discs, one type only if you download it off the Internet.

Personal Computer or PC—Your desktop computer. You'll need one of these (or a laptop) to back up your PDA and generally to install programs to your PDA. Certainly your PDA would be a useful organizer without an associated PC, but the idea of a PDA originated with the thought of two-way communications between the two devices and a means of making some of the PC's data easily portable. It's still a nice arrangement.

PDA or Personal Digital Assistant—Also called handheld computer, sometimes called by its brand name (like "Palm" or "Visor", etc.).

RAM or Random Access Memory—As it pertains to your PDA, this is native or internal memory of your handheld device. It is the memory that you can add to, subtract from, and still save. Databases and other types of software operate this way. Your address book and calendar, for example, are stored in RAM memory so that you can easily make changes and HotSync them between your desktop computer and your PDA.

Reset/Hard Reset—This is much like rebooting your PC. If your PDA inexplicably locks up or sends a "Fatal Error" message, you must reset your handheld. A regular or soft reset is accomplished by pushing a reset pin (or a straightened small paperclip) into the reset hole on the back side of your PDA. This is usually accomplished without the loss of any data. The much more ominous hard reset is a last resort when all else, including the soft reset, fails. For this, you need to hold down the power button of your PDA and perform a reset with a pin in the reset hole at the same time. Unfortunately, this results in the loss of all of your data and all of the programs that you have installed to your PDA. Your device will be restored to the condition in which it came from the factory. You start all over by HotSyncing again. Hopefully, you have backed up your data recently.

ROM or Read Only Memory—As it pertains to your PDA, this is memory that is unchangeable. It may be hardware memory, such as the native operating system in some brands (most notably, HandSpring). It may also refer to memory that is stored in external memory cards. Memory card items are altered, in effect, by your PDA (or you) dragging them back to internal memory, changing them, and then sending them back to external memory. This is often going on behind the scenes, but it is a distinction nonetheless.

Screen Saver—In reference to PDAs, screen savers are thin transparent sheets of film that are applied to the screen of the PDA to protect it from scratches. These usually come in packages of several, custom-sized to fit a certain make and model. When the screen saver gets too scratched, simply peel it off and throw it away. Compare this with a $100+ screen replacement.

Shareware—Software that is readily available and shared with other users. The author usually asks you to voluntarily pay a fee. Let your conscience be your guide. Paying the fee (often $5 to $20) usually nets you extra benefits like free upgrades, no delays at startup, or eliminating pesky reminders that you haven't yet registered the software ("nags").

Silkscreen Buttons—These are the flat, internal buttons that are "printed" on the lower part of the screen of your PDA. These are factory installed on the device and usually number four: launch, menu, find, and calculator. These may vary by device or brand. They may appear at the bottom of the screen or may appear on either side of the Graffiti writing area.

Software—As with your full-sized computer, these are programs that enable your handheld computer to perform functions.

Stylus—The small pen-like device that is used to write on the screen of your PDA. Styli (plural) are designed so that they won't scratch the delicate screen of your PDA. You should only use a stylus when writing on your PDA. Anything else will scratch the screen over time.

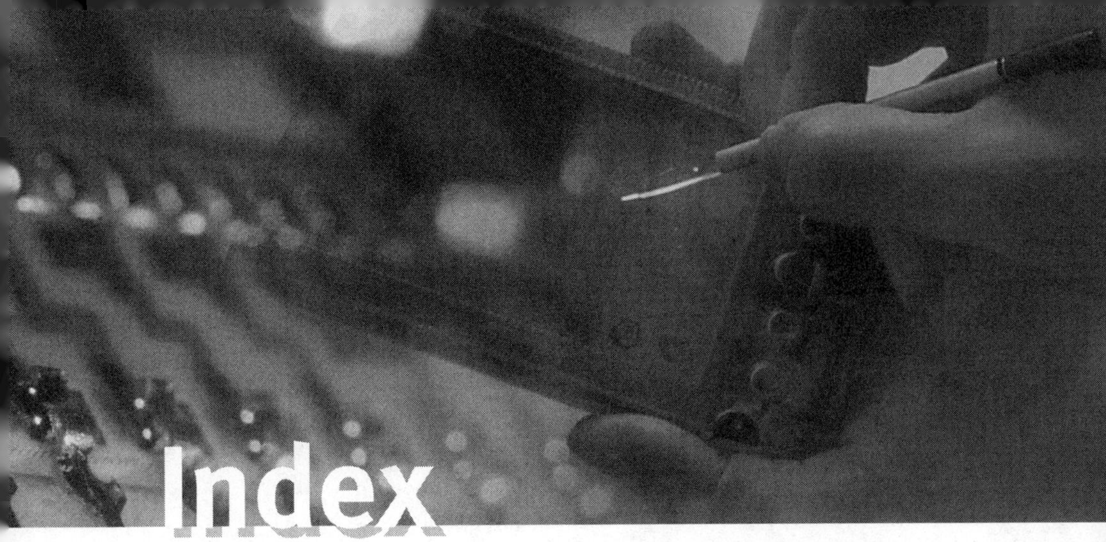

Index

D

E

T

U

V

W

Y

Z